Beyond the Checkup from Birth to Age Four

A PEDIATRICIAN'S GUIDE TO CALM, CONFIDENT PARENTING

Luke Voytas, MD

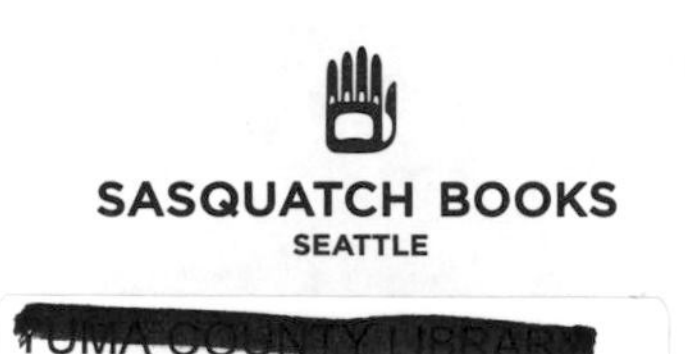

SASQUATCH BOOKS
SEATTLE

Printed in the United States of America

Published by Sasquatch Books

22 21 20 19 18 9 8 7 6 5 4 3 2 1

Editor: Susan Roxborough
Production editor: Em Gale
Design: Bryce de Flamand
Copyeditor: Shari Miranda

Cover photograph: © mapodile | iStock.com
Author photograph: Kat Berbari

Library of Congress Cataloging-in-Publication Data
Names: Voytas, Luke, author.
Title: Beyond the checkup from birth to age four : a pediatrician's guide to calm, confident parenting / Luke Voytas, MD.
Description: Seattle, WA : Sasquatch Books, [2018] | Includes bibliographical references and index.
Identifiers: LCCN 2017061249 | ISBN 9781632171979 (paperback)
Subjects: LCSH: Parenting. | Child rearing. | BISAC: FAMILY & RELATIONSHIPS / Life Stages / Infants & Toddlers. | FAMILY & RELATIONSHIPS / Parenting / General.
Classification: LCC HQ755 .V69 2018 | DDC 649/.1—dc23
LC record available at https://lccn.loc.gov/2017061249

ISBN: 978-1-63217-197-9

Sasquatch Books
1904 Third Avenue, Suite 710
Seattle, WA 98101
(206) 467-4300
SasquatchBooks.com

For Augie and Elsie, always

Table of Contents

Introduction

You are so lucky! You get to have a kid at a time when everything you need to know is right at your literal fingertips. Diaper rash? Fussiness? Question about potty training? BAM! A five-second Google search gives you instant answers—actually, about ten thousand of them. Then you get to pick the one that works best for *you*. If you like judgy or preachy answers, or occasionally enjoy feeling a touch of shame, you're really in luck. And you have social media as a backup, where you don't even *have* to ask a question to get help. Just watch as formerly laid-back family members and friends turn into authoritative health experts!

All right, enough sarcasm—but you see the paradox of being new parents today. For your parents it was simple: listen to Grandma, trust advertisers, and occasionally thumb through the tattered copy of Dr. Spock's baby book. But now we know that a lot of the things your parents did to you are illegal or cause cancer! *You* have access to all the material ever created on parenting but probably come away anxious from that mess of information. This makes it hard to feel confident about what you're doing for your kid! What information is good? Who can you trust? If you're Googling and asking friends online to figure out why your toddler has had a tummy ache for three weeks, you're going to narrow it down to leukemia, constipation, celiac disease, gluten allergy, gluten intolerance, or gluten sensitivity. Not very comforting. And no matter what you do, you're often going to feel *judged*, sometimes in a snarky way and sometimes in an earnest "I just want to help you be a better parent" way that's just as infuriating.

I think you deserve to be a more confident parent, and I think I can help. I've been a general pediatrician for thirteen years and have worked with thousands of new parents. I see them wide-eyed with their newborns in the hospital and get to watch month by month as they grow into calm, confident parents who handle the chaos of toddlerhood like pros. Helping them to develop that confidence is 90 percent of my job (9 percent is playing with your baby, and 1 percent is getting peed on). That *doesn't* happen when I give you handouts or preach to you. I could give you a flyer on feeding, for example, that says, "Make sure to give your child three to five servings of fruits and vegetables a day." Terrific stuff—until your eighteen-month-old smacks those veggies off the table and onto your drapes. *That's* where the real conversation begins. I can't give a one-size-fits-all answer to help your kid sleep better either. As a parent of two young kids myself, I know that it depends on your schedule, your child's personality, the layout of your home, and whether he's prone to pooping on himself at night. I've struggled through most of the topics in this book with my own kids—the sleep deprivation, the meltdowns, the poopy diapers . . . the endless poopy diapers—and am a better pediatrician because of it.

All the technology in the world can't replace a *conversation*. Raising a kid is rarely black or white, and thoughtful chats are how we muddle through the gray. Conversations are relaxed, authentic, and one of the best ways to ease your anxiety as a parent. But I only have fifteen minutes every few months to help you sort through the nonstop barrage of opinions that is thrown at you every day. That has always frustrated me. I wrote this book to extend that discussion and give you some support until your next visit.

We'll begin with what science tells us—lots of interesting studies on kids *just like yours* that try to answer questions about behavior, eating, and sleep. Being able to distinguish good evidence from bad is more important than ever, and we doctors don't do a good enough job of helping you with that. Research is never the final answer for your kid, but it's a good place to start.

ON THE SOURCES CITED IN THIS BOOK

I've cited seventy-one sources for this book out of hundreds that I reviewed. Most are articles from reputable peer-reviewed journals (this means that articles written by experts are reviewed by other experts before they are published). You'll notice that many are from *Pediatrics*, probably the most respected and influential journal in my field. Most studies are recent and use large sample sizes. Whenever possible I've tried to use research that is randomized (participants randomly assigned to different study groups), double-blinded (neither the researchers nor the participants know which group they're in), and placebo-controlled (one group gets a "sham" treatment, which should have no effect), because these factors make conclusions stronger. I've favored studies that are *prospective* (following a group of subjects over time) over those that are *retrospective* (looking backward and depending on parents' recall of events.) That all being said, you can't experiment on young kids as readily as adults, so some of the studies are not perfect. I also use a lot of data from the Centers for Disease Control and Prevention (CDC), which keeps meticulous and trusted statistics on everything from vaccines to sugar consumption.

I give brief descriptions of many of the studies in the text but have written expanded summaries for some of the more important ones in the endnotes. I hope that you feel empowered to use the references to look up additional information on any topics you find interesting.

Then, we'll admit that the work of raising a kid is mostly off the map, without any studies to tell us what to do. We'll acknowledge that there's no precisely perfect way to do things, so we'll just be reasonable and flexible. Like me, you might have pretty strong opinions about some of these issues, like vaccines, sleep training, and discipline. Our opinions might be different. That's okay. I give you the best information I can, and then I trust you to do what's best for *your* kid. Either way, the goal is for you to be a more confident parent.

We'll use the normal "well check" schedule through age four as a framework to talk about issues that come up around those ages. We'll be touching on things like sleep and eating in almost every chapter (since they are going to dominate your life), but other topics, like childproofing or starting preschool, might only come up in one. I have included frequently asked questions at the end of each chapter about both serious and silly things that tend to come up a lot. And the answer is usually going to be "It's normal!"

Your child is going to get sick (it's simply unavoidable), so in the last part of the book we'll explore some of the more common illnesses you might see over the next few years. I have tried to make this stuff easier to remember by providing a lighthearted case study about a particular kid for each example. I want you to know *exactly* what to do when your kid wakes up with crazy vomiting or a fever of 104 degrees Fahrenheit and no other symptoms. I want you to be confident, and Dr. Google isn't going to make that happen.

This book is by no means an exhaustive look at all the issues affecting infants and toddlers, but it does dive into the most common and concerning topics that I talk about with families every day. I hope you'll find it easy enough to just read through, to use as a reference, or to help prepare for checkups with your doctor. I'm also counting on you to be a bit sleep-deprived (a pretty safe bet for new parents), because then my jokes will seem funnier than they really are.

ARE WE CRAZY? WHAT ARE WE GETTING OURSELVES INTO? ARE WE GOING TO BE OKAY?

Kind of. You have no idea. And you'll be fine.

The Final Preparations

Morning sickness is a distant memory. All of a sudden you're at thirty weeks—this is really going to happen! You're excited, anxious, and occasionally horrified that you have no idea what you're doing. First of all, realize that *all* new parents (even pediatricians!) have those thoughts. Soak it up! Think about what your baby's going to look like, the things you want to teach him, the sports she might play, all the ways you want him to be better than you. That's the good stuff. But there are a few business items you need to take care of too, so let's begin.

FINDING THE RIGHT DOCTOR FOR YOUR BABY

Your choice of doctor certainly isn't permanent—plenty of parents switch to find the right fit as their child grows—but it pays to put some time into what could be an eighteen-year relationship. You're going to trust this person to handle your baby and to make sure everything is okay with her. You'll laugh with this doctor, brag to her, and probably even cry in front of her. Sometimes you won't see her for a year, and then you'll see her four times in a month. You might feel like you don't have a whole lot of info to go on to make such a big decision other than online reviews, but let me give you a few additional pointers.

Ideally, you should try to find a pediatrician for your baby. No other provider has more training to take care of your kid. After four years of medical school, general pediatricians do three more years of residency where they spend all of their time (a *lot* of time) taking care of kids. Kids are usually pretty healthy and straightforward, but you want someone who can diagnose the rare stuff too, and a pediatrician can do that. Family doctors can also take terrific care of your kid; just make sure you find one who sees a lot of children, since doctors' experience can vary widely.

The best way to find the best doctor is to talk with other parents—no online review can replace a personal recommendation. Talk to your friends and coworkers, especially people with similar views on parenting as you—people you think of as good parents. If you're new in town, I strongly suggest hooking up with a parents' (or moms' or dads') group. There are really strong parent networks all over the country, and I think they're a terrific resource. More on that later.

There are a few other factors to consider. Some doctors are very popular, and there's probably a reason for that. But it also means their practices are jam-packed, so you may have to wait longer to get an appointment. Some parents feel it's important to have a pediatrician who's the same gender as their child. I know a number of families who even divide up their children between doctors by gender. This is always welcome, but realize that there aren't many gender-specific concerns over the first ten years. And, while a good doctor can tackle any male or female problem until age eighteen, teenagers can always switch to a same-gender provider if they are more comfortable.

Even when you pick a doctor, remember that it's not set in stone. You need to keep evaluating that "fit." Do you get along well with the doctor? Does she mesh with your personality? Some parents, for example, are more anxious than others and worry constantly about whether or not they're doing the right things for their baby. That can make the first year a bit more stressful than it needs to be. These parents might benefit from having a pediatrician who is calm and relaxed, someone who reassures them that they're doing a great job.

Does the doctor make you feel comfortable? Do you feel like you can be honest with him and not be judged? Everyone's schedule is busy and tight, but you shouldn't feel that. Do you feel rushed, or does the doctor take the time to answer all of your questions? Is he interacting more with the computer or your kid? Above all, ask yourself this simple question when you walk out of the office: Do you feel good about your kid and how you're doing as parents? A good pediatrician will make you feel that way even when he has to share concerns about your child.

Finally, don't be afraid to switch doctors within the same practice. This happens all the time in my clinic, and no one takes it personally. You pick a doctor you don't know well and like her just fine, but maybe you come in for a sick visit with another doctor, and it's just a great interaction. It's okay to make the change! It's too important a relationship to worry about offending anyone.

PICKING THE RIGHT CLINIC

You're also choosing a medical practice along with the doctor. These come in all shapes and sizes, and you will want to do some homework. Many parents just take their child to the closest clinic, but driving five more minutes for the right clinic can be well worth it. How do you find out more about the practice? Some clinics allow you to meet and "interview" the doctor before baby comes. Others host open houses where you can take a tour. Websites can give you a lot of information as well. Here are some questions to consider:

- What kind of hours do they have? Do they open early in the morning and have extended hours in the evening? Things happen on the weekends—do they have Saturday or Sunday hours for sick visits? Urgent care clinics play an important role, but it's a plus to see *your* doctor if you're worried about an ear infection on a Saturday.

- How many patients per day do doctors usually see there? You might be surprised how much this can vary. Doctors can see anywhere from fifteen to forty or more patients per day. A busy doctor can be efficient and take good care of his or her patients, but a doctor who sees fewer patients simply has more time to spend with you.

- Is it easy to get a same-day appointment when your child is sick? As adults, most people don't expect this availability. For your child, you *should* expect it.

- Will doctors from that practice see your newborn in the hospital? Increasingly, more facilities are using pediatric hospitalists, pediatricians whose specialty is taking care of newborns and kids only when they're in the hospital. They will provide excellent care—but it can be nice seeing *your* doctor in the hospital.

- What kind of ancillary services are available at the clinic? Do they have a lab and radiology on-site or nearby? Are they located next to a hospital?

- Who will be seeing your baby at visits? Will it usually be your child's doctor, or is there another provider who does many of the sick visits? Does the doctor always work with the same nurse or medical assistant? This individual will interact with your kid a lot while settling you into the exam room, and it can really be nice to see a familiar face (or mildly alarming for your kid to see the same face that always gives her shots, I suppose!).

- Can you call anytime? And who will be taking your call? You should be able to get ahold of someone twenty-four hours a day, seven days a week. This could be advice nurses at the clinic, the doctor himself, or a highly trained pediatric nurse triage line (often used by practices to field routine calls in the middle of the night).

WHAT TO BUY—KEEP IT SIMPLE!

It's baby shower time (which apparently is a co-ed thing now, as my wife tells me). There is a *lot* of stuff out there. So what should you buy? *As little as possible!*

Companies know that you're anxious to buy *anything* that might help your baby. And they want to sell you all those things! There are a few items that are really crucial, and then there is plenty more that is just expensive clutter. Here are some things that I think are important:

A BASSINET. This is your baby's ideal sleeping place for the first few months—a little mini crib right next to your bed so she's easy to find in your sleep-deprived state. Most play yards (a magical little fold-up crib that you can take with you on trips) have a bassinet attachment for the top that works perfectly fine.

A CRIB. Remember that all cribs on the market since 2011 meet strict safety guidelines. So if you like the way something looks or how it matches your wainscoting, great—but you should also feel comfortable getting something cheap or used from a trusted source.

A BABY CARRIER. I recommend a style like Baby Bjorn or Ergobaby—one that carries your baby in front of you facing either direction. This is going to give you your hands back someday, and it's good to have hands. Carriers are pricey, so don't hesitate to go secondhand.

A MONITOR. These can get pretty over the top, even syncing up with your phone and letting you check your baby's vital signs, but something basic will let you know when your baby is upset and needs some help. You'll travel with this thing and get plenty of use out of it.

A CAR SEAT. Notice I did not say a top-of-the-line car seat. Parents often tell me proudly that they got the most expensive one available. It feels good to know you've bought the best for your baby, and your baby's safety is serious business. But as with cribs, car seats all have to meet some pretty strict safety guidelines. The cheap ones will work awesomely. Your baby won't miss the three cupholders and the shiatsu massage capability. (However, this is the one time to avoid buying used: You can't be sure of the car seat's history, and they need to be replaced after even a minor car accident.) Two quick hints:

1. You can buy an infant carrier that protects a child weighing up to twenty-two or thirty pounds. A lot of parents buy the thirty-pound seat thinking that it's a better value because they can use it longer. But by the time your baby is twenty-two pounds you're not going to be lifting that thing in and out of the car anymore and it's going to be time to get a bigger-kid car seat (still facing the back, of course). Buying the thirty-pound seat just means more money, more bulk, and more weight to carry around for the first year.

2. Having a car seat brand that clicks into your stroller is pretty nice. It saves a lot of time and prevents waking babies during transfers.

A STROLLER. There are as many different types of strollers as there are types of parents, so which one to choose really depends on your lifestyle. I think it's important to get out and about with your baby, so I'm partial to jogging strollers. They have really big wheels and a suspension system, are easy to maneuver, and often have attachments that let you snap your infant carrier right into them. They're expensive, but you can save a lot of money by getting a used one and then selling it (for not much less) when your kiddos get older. Many brands also make a model for two kids, with which you'll utterly dominate the neighborhood sidewalks. I think it's useful to have a cheap umbrella stroller as well for traveling.

AS MANY USED CLOTHES AS POSSIBLE. I really mean this. You will be *happy* to spend money on fancy new clothes for your baby. She'll look impossibly cute in all of them, and it will make you feel good. But your baby doesn't care. And babies grow fast! You'll have the inevitable experience of finding a super cute pair of pinstriped overalls in the bottom of the dresser with the tags still on that your baby has already outgrown. Trust me, nothing feels better than dumping a few bags of baby clothes on a friend with a newborn, so take advantage of that. Your baby will bring more love than clutter into your life, but just by a little bit.

AN INFANT SWING. This is my luxury item, a splurge (look for a gently used one at consignment shops). But wow, having a portable place where your baby is calm, and being able to use your arms—your actual *arms*—for one or two hours? That may be priceless. Pretty nice for the first three months.

THE COST OF KIDS

According to the USDA, the average middle-income parents are projected to spend $233,610 to raise one child born in 2015 to age seventeen (um, that doesn't even include college). That's a lot of money! The top three expenses were housing, childcare/education, and food. Costs depend on where you live and your income level, so check out the USDA's calculator to get a better estimate for your kid.[1]

In closing, you really don't have to buy much for your baby. There's so much used baby stuff floating around in mint condition, and usually those with older kids are happy to get rid of it—you probably have a few friends who would love to offload (does anybody want a not-so-gently used retro play kitchen? Anybody?). And remember, college is expensive. It might be ridiculous to even think about it when your kid is still pooping on herself, but the $100 you can save by holding off on the bamboo-fiber wipe warmer today could be $1,000 toward college in eighteen years.

A FEW OTHER CONSIDERATIONS

It's important to think ahead of time about vaccines for people who might spend a lot of time around your baby. Mom should get a Tdap vaccine with each pregnancy. The "P" stands for pertussis (also known as whooping cough). Infants can't get vaccinated for this until two months, and it can be a devastating illness for them. Dad and other caregivers should also get a Tdap if they have never had one. If it's flu season (October to March), encourage everyone who will come in contact with your baby to get a flu shot, because she can't receive one until six months.

You'll also want to stock your medicine cabinet for the inevitable sniffles and discomforts that come about in the first couple years. Don't worry, you can make plenty of space in there by throwing out all your primping products: you'd actually have to *go out* over the next few years to care about how you look when you go out. Here are the essentials I recommend you have on hand:

ACETAMINOPHEN (TYLENOL). This is the heavy hitter for the first six months. Don't use it for ordinary fussiness, but if your baby develops a fever and acts cranky, it can be a lifesaver. Also, if your child gets vaccines and seems upset later in the day, it can help. If your baby's younger than two months old, make sure to touch base with your doctor before you give it. Hint: Liquid acetaminophen only comes in one concentration now (160 mg/5 ml), but it's packaged separately for infants and children. The infant product is about the same price for way less volume, so just get the children's one.

IBUPROFEN (MOTRIN, ADVIL). You can't use ibuprofen until your baby is six months old, but then it becomes precious. Like acetaminophen, it will help with your baby's fever or pain. But only ibuprofen will help with inflammation, so it's an excellent choice for "inflamed" things like sore throats and ears. Plus, it lasts for six or more hours as opposed to acetaminophen's four.

DIPHENHYDRAMINE (BENADRYL). This is an antihistamine—histamine is the main chemical in your body that makes you itchy, and it kind of goes crazy if you're having an allergic reaction. The syrup only comes in one concentration (12.5 mg/5 ml), and you want to have it on hand for an allergic reaction, hives, or other types of itching. The package will probably say for ages two and up, but it's certainly fine after six months. Call your doctor for the right dose. Note that it can make your child a bit drowsy.

HYDROCORTISONE 1% CREAM. This is a super-weak steroid that you can buy over the counter. Steroid is a scary word, but don't be afraid of this product. A few applications of hydrocortisone will help most rashes that are bothering your baby but not responding to simple moisturizers.

VASELINE/AQUAPHOR. These thick ointments are barriers. They are great to use for dry skin, facial rashes, and to protect the skin folds of chubby six-month-olds from getting irritated. Aquaphor is just Vaseline with some lanolin added to make it a bit more spreadable.

EUCERIN/CETAPHIL/CERAVE CREAM. These are thick lotions that rub completely into the skin and don't have any dyes or perfumes in them. They don't act as a barrier but are great for dry skin and not as goopy. Experiment to find one that you like.

DIAPER CREAM. There are countless brands, but you basically want two types on hand. First, a good maximum-strength zinc oxide cream (e.g., Desitin or Boudreaux's Butt Paste), which is a workhorse that is great for moderate and severe diaper rashes. Second, A+D ointment, which is a little thinner but easier to work with and good for mild rashes or daily prevention.

CLOTRIMAZOLE 1% CREAM (LOTRIMIN). This is a great general antifungal cream for diaper and skin fungal infections, which are more common than you think.

It's Go Time!

BIRTH AND THE FIRST FEW DAYS

I'm excited for you to see your baby and hear him cry for the first time. It's unreal, and your heart is going to do things it's never done before. The delivery room can be rather overwhelming (don't lock those knees, Dad—passing out is such a cliché!) with a bunch of people in scrubs buzzing around. If all goes according to plan, those nurses and doctors will check your baby but then quickly hand him over to Mom. Skin-to-skin time is really a priority: Babies who go right up against their mom's chest have a more stable heart rate and blood pressure, and better breathing. They maintain a more stable blood sugar and body temperature. They even latch better and are more successful at breastfeeding over the first year. There's been substantial progress in this area over the past decade. The most important thing used to be doctors like me taking over the care of your newborn, but now it's the bond between you and your baby. Within the first few hours, the nurses will ask permission to give three medicines to your baby:

VITAMIN K INJECTION. This is the most important "medical" thing done after birth in my opinion, and it should be a no-brainer for you. Vitamin K is crucial to prevent bleeding, but newborns have very low levels. Breast milk doesn't have much vitamin K in it either. The CDC reports[2] that one in sixty to one in 250 newborns will develop bleeding due to vitamin K deficiency, which can be devastating if it occurs in the brain. Late bleeding can happen up until six months old—it is rarer but often more severe, and eighty-one times more likely in babies who don't get the vitamin K shot. There are some untrue rumors circulating around the internet that a vitamin K shot can cause cancer, contain toxic preservatives, or lead to infection. Some parents also want to give it by mouth instead of by injection, but that method doesn't work as well. In my seventeen years of schooling and practice, I have *never* seen a side effect from the vitamin K shot, and I think it's really important for your baby.

HEPATITIS B VACCINE. Hepatitis B is a virus that attacks your liver. It's pretty common in adults (including pregnant moms!), most of whom have no symptoms and don't know they have it. Doctors usually test moms for it during pregnancy, but the testing isn't perfect. Newborns can also get the disease from other caregivers over the first few months. By giving this safe vaccine routinely at birth, we significantly cut down the number of infants who get this lifelong disease. The second dose is usually given at two months.

ERYTHROMYCIN OINTMENT. This is a safe antibiotic ointment that the nurses will apply to your baby's eyes one time. It helps prevent severe eye infections in the first few weeks after birth due to maternal chlamydia or gonorrhea, as well as other bacteria such as staph.

A doctor, usually a pediatrician, will come to examine your baby and talk with you within the first twenty-four hours. You'll see the labor and delivery nurses a lot more often. They are a treasure trove of knowledge and will likely do more than anyone to jumpstart your confidence as a parent. There are a few things that both the doctors and nurses are going to be watching for:

HOW IS YOUR BABY EATING? Remember—and this is very important—your baby is born not needing much food for the first few days. Babies are born with an extra fluid reserve—I like to think of it as a little survival backpack—that they can live off of for two to three days until Mom's milk comes in. Some babies will latch well and breastfeed right away. Others will take a while, like a full day or two. I really want to emphasize that your baby is built to get through those first days even when feeding is a struggle! So hang in there! Most hospitals have lactation specialists, and I tell *everyone* to take advantage of them. Even if feeding is going well, they will always have some great tips to make your life easier. The staff will also keep track of your baby's weight. All babies lose weight for the first few days; the hope is that they lose less than 10 percent of their birth weight before they start gaining again. If it's near that mark, doctors might suggest supplementing with any extra milk Mom is able to pump, formula, or donor milk (carefully screened and usually only an option while in the hospital), until Mom's milk more fully comes in.

IS YOUR BABY PEEING AND POOPING? The doctors will want your baby to pee and poop at least once in the first twenty-four hours, which tells them that his kidneys and intestines are working. The first few black tarry poops are called meconium, and your baby is preloaded with it—it has nothing to do with what he's eating yet. Be prepared for the pees to slow down on days two and three (as few as one or two a day), when your baby has used up most of his reserves but isn't getting much from Mom yet. Once your milk does come in, your baby should start peeing six or more times a day.

PINK PEE!

You might notice that your baby's pee leaves a pink or orange stain on the diaper at times over the first few days. Don't panic, it's not blood! It's just uric acid crystals that form in your baby's urine when it gets a bit concentrated (usually before Mom's milk has come in), and it's totally normal.

HOW JAUNDICED IS YOUR BABY? All babies get a little bit jaundiced. Jaundice just means that an increased amount of a chemical called bilirubin is found in your baby's blood. We make a fuss over it because if the level gets really high, it can enter your baby's brain and cause some permanent damage called *kernicterus*. A few factors can increase your baby's chance of having a problem with jaundice. These include prematurity, swelling or bruising on his head, and Mom's blood not agreeing with his blood. A nurse will check your baby's level through the skin with a fancy little light sensor or by a blood test when he is about twenty-four hours old. Fortunately, there's a pretty easy treatment for jaundice. They can put your baby under some bright UV lights that actually break down the bilirubin in his skin. This is called phototherapy.

Jaundice makes your baby look yellow, and the higher the level of bilirubin, the more yellow your baby will look. It also weirdly creeps from the head down the body the more severe it gets. So his face and eyes can look yellow at pretty low levels. If jaundice is going to be a problem, we'll usually know it in the first four or five days, but breastfed babies can have noticeable jaundice that lingers for weeks. This "breast milk jaundice" almost never causes issues, and your pediatrician will keep an eye on it.

ARE THERE ANY SIGNS OF INFECTION? Infection is pretty rare, but it happens—and doctors don't like to take any chances. About one in four moms test positive for group B strep (GBS) bacteria a few weeks before delivery, and their babies have a higher risk of serious infection. Your obstetrician can minimize this by giving you a couple doses of antibiotics before delivery. If the birth happens quickly without enough time for the antibiotics, your baby might have to be observed for a full forty-eight hours. Your baby's vital signs will be followed closely as well—his heart rate, respiratory rate, and temperature. This can give doctors a clue if an infection is starting, and sometimes bloodwork or a few days of antibiotics will be recommended.

HOW IS YOUR BABY'S BLOOD SUGAR? Some babies are born with a higher risk for having low blood sugar (or glucose) over the first few days. This includes babies who are kind of big, kind of small, or whose moms had gestational diabetes or received certain medicines during labor. If their blood sugar gets too low, babies can get jittery or even have seizures. So doctors check it before and after the first few feeds (by poking their poor little heels) and try to supplement a bit if it's getting low. For the few babies that still struggle, the backup is giving sugar through an IV for a short period of time. Once your baby has had stable sugars for a few feeding cycles, he's usually out of the woods.

HOW DOES YOUR BABY LOOK? Babies aren't born looking like the Gerber baby. Of course they're precious right away, but sometimes their appearance can be downright shocking. One of the jobs of the nurses and doctors is to reassure you that all the weird-looking stuff is normal—except in the rare cases where it isn't. So let's talk about some of the appearances you might not be expecting:

> **CONE-SHAPED HEADS.** The bones that make up your baby's skull are designed to be molded to help that big noggin get through the birth canal. But it can literally be a cone, startling even the most laid-back new parents. You might also feel a bunch of ridges on your baby's head, which are just where the skull bones come together. Watching the head reshape itself over the first three days gives you a great sense of how resilient your baby is.
>
> **MUSHY HEADS.** Many babies who have endured difficult deliveries will have fluid that collects under a certain part of their scalp. This feels kind of "boggy" to the touch and can make the head look pretty lumpy. These bumps resolve on their own within a

few days or weeks (depending on which level of the scalp the fluid is trapped under). It doesn't affect the brain at all.

PURPLE HANDS AND FEET. One nice thing our bodies do for us is clamp down our blood vessels in our hands and feet when we get cold. This keeps the blood in the middle of our bodies to keep the important stuff warm. But this system is a little bit twitchy in babies, so their blood vessels can randomly clamp down until they look like they're wearing purple socks and gloves. This is always okay and doesn't mean that your baby is too cold or low on oxygen.

SWOLLEN EYELIDS AND STUFFY NOSES. The eyes and nose take a lot of pressure on the way out, and they both swell up quite easily. So don't be alarmed if your baby's eyelids are so puffy that he can hardly open his eyes on the first day. The nose is just mushy cartilage and will recover in no time, but the swelling can create some congestion and snorty breathing sounds.

BLOODSHOT EYES. It's attention-grabbing, but lots of babies have bright red lines in the white of their eyes, usually right along the edge of the iris (colored part). These are just tiny broken blood vessels from the pressure of being born. They aren't painful and go away during the first few weeks.

EYE BOOGERS. Over the next few months you might see stringy white goop at the inside corners of your baby's eyes. It might extend along the bottom of the eyelid as well. This is usually caused by a clogged tear duct. We all have little ducts in the inside corners of our eyes that drain old tears and residue. In babies these ducts are tiny. You can help by wiping away the goop with a warm washcloth and massaging with your (clean!) pinky from the inner part of the eye down along the edge of the nose. If the goop comes back every hour or the eye turns red after a few days, that could be a sign of infection.

The nurses will also get a few drops of blood from your baby's heel and send it off to test for rare diseases like cystic fibrosis and phenylketonuria (PKU). The specific diseases tested vary from state to state, but they are mostly rare illnesses with bad outcomes that can be prevented if we know about them early. Your pediatrician may repeat them at the two-week visit.

Your baby will also probably get a hearing test—this is usually done with some small headphones while your baby is sleeping. And if he does not pass the first time, there is a great chance that he will later. Finally, the medical staff might do a test where they check the oxygen level in your baby's arms and legs to make sure that his heart is pumping equally everywhere.

EARLY SPITTING UP AND GAGGING

When your baby is a few weeks old, he'll spit up because he's getting a lot of milk from you. But in the hospital, most spitting up is caused by taking a big gulp of amniotic fluid on the way out. Babies can spit this light yellow fluid up over the first one to two days. You can often tell when it's coming because he'll make urpy gulps just beforehand. Parents have two concerns about this.

First, when newborns spit up it can often trigger the gag reflex. Your baby has a vicious gag reflex, which is awesome. If anything besides air even gets close to his airway, his throat muscles clamp down like a trap. But even though this *prevents* your baby from choking, it can sure look like he *is* choking rather than gagging. He might cough, sputter, and not breathe for twenty seconds.

His face might turn red or purple. His eyes might water. It's all pretty alarming. But try to stay calm, turn him onto his side, rub his back, and just wait for those muscles to relax. He'll be okay.

Second, parents know that it's safest for newborns to sleep on their backs in a bassinet. But they worry about what might happen if he spits up while he's on his back. What if you don't wake up? Again, your baby is *tough*. He'll just turn his head to the side, and those throat muscles will pop that spit-up out. No problem. Plus, you're not going to be sleeping *that* deeply anyway . . . for quite some time. Sorry.

WHY THE SECOND NIGHT IS ROUGHER THAN THE FIRST

Being born is hard work. Your baby has some serious adrenaline going, and then he's going to crash from that adrenaline. So babies often sleep pretty hard for the first twenty-four hours. You're still going to try to feed him every few hours, but he's using that extra fluid in his survival backpack. The few drops of colostrum he *does* get from Mom give his immune system an early boost. By the second night, however, he'll start to get *feisty*. He'll cry more and may want to cluster his feeds as often as every hour. This is exhausting for you, but it's a good thing! All that sucking will bring Mom's milk in quicker and help your baby to gain some weight back.

A WORD ON BREASTFEEDING

I encourage you to breastfeed—at least give it a try. It can be a bit daunting, but remember that it's normal for breastfeeding to be frustrating, confusing, and painful for the first few days or even weeks. You know that it's the best nutrition for your baby, but you deserve to know the specifics of why. I don't think most people realize how massive the benefits are, not just for the first year but for conditions that could affect your child's whole life! Here's what the American Academy of Pediatrics has found:[3]

- Breastfeeding significantly lowers rates of illnesses both during infancy and later in life. For example, breastfed babies have:
    - Up to 40 percent lower rates of asthma if breastfed exclusively for at least three months
    - 50 percent lower rates of ear infections if breastfed exclusively for at least three months
    - 63 percent lower rates of colds if breastfed exclusively for at least six months
    - 72 percent lower rates of lung infections if breastfed exclusively for at least four months
    - 24 percent lower rates of obesity for *any* breastfeeding
    - 36 percent lower rates of SIDS (sudden infant death syndrome) for *any* breastfeeding
    - 40 percent lower rates of type 2 diabetes for *any* breastfeeding
    - 64 percent lower rates of gastroenteritis (stomach viruses) for *any* breastfeeding
- Children who were breastfed as infants seem to have slightly higher intelligence scores when they're older, even when researchers take into account differences in education, age, and socioeconomic status between breastfeeding and formula groups.
- Breastfeeding benefits seem to be particularly strong in premature infants.
- Mothers who breastfeed have decreased rates of postpartum depression, type 2 diabetes, heart disease, and certain types of cancer.

- Cost is certainly not the most important factor, but you will also save a significant amount of money by not having to buy formula or miss as much work due to your baby's illnesses.

Medical reasons to avoid breastfeeding are rare. A mom with HIV or an infant with galactosemia (a rare metabolic condition) are the only firm contraindications. Moms with untreated tuberculosis or active herpes lesions at the breast shouldn't nurse, but they can give pumped milk. Marijuana gets highly concentrated in breast milk and could potentially affect brain development, so breastfeeding moms should avoid using it. Most common medications are probably fine to use while breastfeeding, but ask your doctor if you're not sure.

In talking about all of the benefits of breastfeeding, I do worry that I might contribute to the frustration of moms who either choose not to or are unable to breastfeed. Sometimes breastfeeding doesn't work out, or you might feel that it requires so much time that it affects care of your other children or your career. And some women choose not to breastfeed simply because they don't want to. And that's okay. With all these issues, you gather good information, you get the support you need, and in the end you make the best decision for your family. I don't judge that, and it's a good bet that your child's doctor won't either. Your baby is going to be just fine either way.

FORMULA FRENZY

If you do feed your baby formula, how do you pick one? There is some incredible marketing with formula. You'll receive unsolicited samples in the mail and maybe even in the hospital. Formula cans are covered with fancy words like DHA, probiotics, and prebiotics, hinting that *this formula alone* will help your baby be smarter and healthier. Even if money is tight, as a new parent you're eager to give your baby the best. This is why most parents end up using "trusted" name-brand formula.

But I'm telling you to use the *cheapest store-brand formula you can find* (sorry, Similac and Enfamil). Really. Costco, Target, Walgreens, etc. They have exactly the same nutrition and meet the same strict guidelines set by the Food and Drug Administration (FDA) and the American Academy of Pediatrics (AAP). A 2012 study[4] comparing babies' reactions to different formulas suggests that store-brand options are tolerated just as well as the name brands. You can get all the same miracle additives in them as well. The only difference is that they cost up to 50 percent less than the national brands, saving your family hundreds of dollars over the first year. So get rid of that little speck of doubt that you will be somehow compromising your baby's well-being.

BREASTFEEDING TRENDS

Breastfeeding rates have been rising for quite some time in the United States. The CDC's Breastfeeding Report Card for 2016[5] found that 81 percent of newborns start out breastfeeding, compared to only 70 percent in 2000. However, there's a fairly steep drop-off. Only 52 percent of infants were still breastfeeding at six months and just 30 percent at twelve months.

GET ME OUTTA HERE!

If things are going well and you had a vaginal delivery, you'll usually be released from the hospital in under forty-eight hours. If you had a C-section it will usually add an extra day as your baby waits for you to recover. It will then be important for your baby to have a postpartum check two days after you go home, either at the hospital or your pediatrician's office. Some facilities will stretch this to three days, but I'm always more comfortable with two—that gives us a better chance of identifying weight or jaundice problems before they become severe. There may be a lactation specialist available to help you at that time too. If everything looks great at the postpartum check, the next visit will usually be at two weeks with your baby's doctor.

BASIC BABY MAINTENANCE—LESS IS MORE!

You'll soon be at home, settling into a wonderful delirium of feeding, diaper changing, and cuddling. That stuff will become automatic soon enough, but, since your baby doesn't come with a manual, here are some tips on the finer points of caring for your lovebug.

BATHING. Your baby's skin is designed pretty well. Resist the urge to bathe him frequently. He's not really that dirty yet (that will come later with a vengeance). Once or twice a week is perfect. More than that will tend to dry his skin out.

SKIN CARE. Your baby is probably going to get kind of peely over the next two weeks, especially around the ankles, wrists, and stomach. This is just the outer layer of skin that was protecting him from the amniotic fluid. It's now sloughing away and that's totally normal. There's a good healthy layer of skin underneath, so no need to put lotion on it. In fact, try to go easy on the lotion for the next few months—covering your baby with it will make it a bit harder for him to cool himself down.

FINGERNAILS. Parents are *terrified* of cutting baby fingernails! But those little things are razor sharp and babies can accidentally scratch up their faces and eyes. I'm not going to sugarcoat it. Just get in there with an adult nail clipper (I think it's easier to use than the baby versions), hold the finger really firmly, and get it done. If he's wiggly, just do three or four at a time. Infant nails are usually too flimsy to file. And biting them or tearing them could cause infections and is just kind of weird. The worst thing that could ever happen is that you clip a bit of skin on the tip of his finger (which my wife did to *both* of our kids!). Those nails grow fast, so be ready to repeat this every four or five days.

THE UMBILICAL CORD STUMP. Just ignore it. Doctors used to suggest putting rubbing alcohol on it and obsessing over it, but now we know that it takes care of itself and usually falls off between one and two weeks if you keep it dry and leave it alone. For this reason, sponge baths are best until it's gone. Be ready to see some goopy, stinky stuff at the base that almost looks like pus when it is about to fall off. When it finally does, it's normal for the belly button to ooze and cause some stains on the onesie for a few more days. You can clean it with warm water and mild soap while it's draining. If the oozing doesn't stop after a few days, call your doctor.

FAQS

What do we do about fever, and what type of thermometer should we use?

Good question. Fever is a *big deal* before two months of age. Your newborn doesn't have a great barrier yet between his blood and his brain, so infections can get into the brain more easily than for older children. Before two months, a temperature of 100.4 degrees F or higher is an emergency, and you should call your pediatrician or take your baby in right away. The doctor might have to check your baby's blood, urine, and even spinal fluid to rule out any bacterial infections. For most babies, a simple virus is causing the fever, but we don't take chances.

That said, you do *not* have to routinely check your baby's temperature! That will just make you pointlessly nervous—your baby is going to let you know if something's wrong. Nursing moms can usually tell when their baby feels warm, and persistent irritability or poor feedings would also be reasons to check. At this age, a cheap metal-tipped digital thermometer works best. You can start by checking in the armpit, and if it's normal then you're done. If it's in the mid-99s or higher, though, you'll want to get a rectal temperature with the same thermometer. That's always spot-on.

What kind of diapers should we use?

This is totally a personal preference, but here are my two cents. Most people certainly use disposable. The advantages are that they are super convenient, super absorbent, and relatively cheap when you buy them in bulk. Maybe the worst part is the massive amount of waste they generate, which really bothers some people. You could easily go through eighty diapers a week for the first few months. I don't know if it's considered toxic waste, but it's got to be close. Fortunately, a growing number of companies are targeting more environmentally conscious parents by offering biodegradable options.

Cloth diapers are becoming more popular, and fortunately they've come a long way since safety pins were the only protection our parents had against blowouts. There are now waterproof covers that either have a snap-in insert, a loose diaper inside, or a pouch where you insert one. If you wash your own diapers (a *big* job), you would save money over disposable but lose a lot of time and be even further immersed in the world of poop.

My wife and I decided to use a diaper service for our kids, where you keep all the dirty cloth diapers in a big awful bin and they come by and exchange that awfulness for a fresh pile of gleaming white diapers every week. How they get them that clean I don't want to know. The major benefit is that you're being a lot gentler on the environment, and some would argue that you're exposing your baby's skin to fewer chemicals. The diaper services say that you'll save money in the long run and that your kid will potty train earlier because he can feel the moisture against his skin better. I don't think either of these is actually true. Another downside is that they are quite a bit more bulky than disposables. The first time I saw my son in a cloth diaper I remember thinking, "My God, is he going to walk like a *cowboy* if we keep him in those?"

Bottom line? Your choice of diapers is really more of a personal choice than something that will benefit your child. I think cloth is a responsible option that's more practical than ever, but you have to make the best decision for your family.

Should we get our son circumcised?

This is a pretty personal decision, but it's still a question I hear a lot. I never give any recommendation, because it's up to you. The American Academy of Pediatrics issued a statement in 2012[6] that there are some clear benefits to the procedure—decreased rates of urinary tract infections, sexually transmitted diseases (the last thing on your mind right now), and penile or cervical (for partners) cancers. Some parents feel it's important that their son "looks like Daddy," and there may be something to that. I agree with the AAP that these modest health benefits should be acknowledged, but they are not necessarily more important than your religious, ethical, and cultural beliefs. Again, it's a personal decision.

On a practical note, it's often easiest to have the circumcision done while you're still in the hospital. In some places pediatricians do it; in others obstetricians tend to. If you're thinking about getting it done in the hospital, you may want to call to ask about costs and policies. Otherwise, try to make arrangements in the first two or three weeks. After that most doctors won't perform the procedure until one year, and then it becomes more of a "real" surgery.

When should we introduce a bottle?

For breastfeeding moms, it can be really useful for your baby to accept a bottle at some point. Especially if you will be going back to work, want to go out for four or more hours at some point over the next year, or (*gasp*) would love to get five consecutive hours of sleep. I think around one month is a fine time to do this—if it's only on occasion, it's unlikely to threaten breastfeeding at this point or cause any "nipple confusion." I recommend starting with a newborn or "low-flow" nipple as well. You don't want him to down the bottle so quickly that feeding at the breast seems like a chore in comparison. And it's probably best for Dad or someone else to give it rather than Mom since your baby will be more likely to want it straight from the source if it's snuggled up against his face.

Our baby sounds really congested. Does he have a cold already?

Newborns can be very noisy breathers. They have really small nasal passages that can be further irritated and swollen from the pressure during birth. So even just the normal snot we all make every day is enough to plug things up. Some of the spit-up finds its way up to the nose as well. Babies can't blow their noses yet, so all of that gunk just hangs out in there and rattles around. Since babies' breathing is quite irregular already (they can take five breaths in five seconds and then hold their breath for the next ten seconds), this can make it seem like he's struggling to breathe sometimes. The best way to tell if he's okay is always through feeding. When babies feed they *have* to breathe through their noses. If he can stay latched on for minutes at a time, you know he's getting enough air through his nose, no matter how noisy it is.

Breastfeeding has been pretty tough these first few days—it's painful and our baby isn't latching that well. The lactation nurse said he might be tongue-tied. Can we do something about that?

Where I live and work, there has been an absolute tongue-tie *frenzy* over the past few years. It has gotten to the point where most moms struggling with breastfeeding over the first few weeks (so, a *lot* of moms) are told by someone that their baby might be tongue-tied. Let's try to demystify it a little bit and be reasonable.

First, what does it mean to be tongue- or lip-tied? It means that your baby has a harder time moving her tongue or lips because of how they are attached to the other structures in her mouth. There are three types you might hear about.

1. ANTERIOR TONGUE-TIE. If you roll the tip of your tongue back in your mouth, you'll see a little thin pink strand of tissue that anchors the middle front of your tongue to the floor of your mouth. In some babies this strand (called a *frenulum*) attaches almost at the tip of the tongue. This can prevent them from sticking their tongue out past the edge of their lower lip. These tongues tend to be heart-shaped when babies stick them out since the middle is anchored down.

   The attachment can be a problem because babies need to stick their tongue out to pull back on the nipple. Tongue-tied babies tend to smack up and down when feeding instead, which is painful for Mom and not very effective at getting milk. These tongue-ties can be legit. A small but well-done 2011 study determined that getting them clipped can improve breastfeeding as well as reduce pain for the mother.[7] And fortunately, the procedure is simple and doesn't require anesthesia. Talk to your pediatrician if you're worried.

2. POSTERIOR TONGUE-TIE. This is the one that's gone a bit off the rails. At the base of your tongue you have tissue that anchors your tongue to the floor of your mouth. Like anything else, there is a spectrum of how mobile tongues are. Some people can touch their nose with the tip of their tongue and some can't get close. Despite this natural variation, some doctors and even dentists have started to perform a more significant procedure where they cut some of that tissue at the base of the tongue with a scalpel or laser.

   I see lots of parents who have had this done to their baby, and most of them feel that it has helped. But the placebo effect is strong! There just isn't any high-quality evidence available that cutting the tissue actually benefits babies. Plus it can cause some scarring and is an expensive procedure not covered by insurance. Maybe in ten years that will be different. Feelings run pretty hot on this issue, so make the best decision for your baby. But remember that desperate parents and a strong placebo effect can create a vacuum for poor science and false hope to move in.

3. UPPER LIP-TIE. This is the little string of tissue you see when you flip up your upper lip. It holds the lip to your gum. There's absolutely no good evidence that this routinely affects breastfeeding. It sometimes needs to be cut for braces or other dental reasons when your child is older.

In our family, boys born in the first half of the year usually have green eyes, and blue eyes seem to skip generations in girls. Everyone with a single-syllable name has brown. What color are my baby's eyes going to be?

I have no idea. And I have no idea why people are obsessed with this, but it's one of the most common questions I get. I usually furrow my brow and take a serious look into your baby's eyes before I make a random declaration (I kind of enjoy that). But the reality is that eye color is not necessarily set until about a year, and I guarantee that your baby's eyes will be lovely no matter what.

Two Weeks

The last two weeks have been a total blur. Day and night are no longer distinct entities. You are developing muscle memory to change diapers while half-asleep. You're starting to realize that your baby is really good at letting you know what she needs—and that's a whole lot right now. When you slog out to the store for essentials, you feel as if you're crawling out of the woods after being lost for months. But you're also starting to feel a bit more confident. You're realizing that she's not as fragile as you had feared—and, hey, you're kind of good at this whole parenting thing. Now that you know you can survive, it's time to lift your chin up and look ahead a bit. There's plenty to talk about.

WHAT YOUR BABY SHOULD BE DOING NOW

The first thing I look at before heading into the room with a two-week-old is weight. Ideally, your baby should at least be back to her birth weight by this time. This tells me two things—that your milk supply is sufficient and that your baby is capable of getting it. But don't panic if she's not quite there yet. If she lost a lot of weight initially but is now gaining at a good rate, that's just fine. Otherwise your pediatrician will work with you on a plan to make sure that she thrives. This could just mean another follow-up appointment in a few days or supplementing with extra milk to ensure that she gets enough.

There are many ways to supplement, but it's crucial to preserve all the breastfeeding progress you've made. When I feel that a baby is struggling to get the milk she needs, I encourage starting every feeding at the breast but stopping before she gets exhausted (usually no more than twenty-five minutes). I then recommend offering a bottle of either pumped milk or formula as a "top-off." Then she is followed closely to make sure that she is *capable* of gaining weight when offered enough calories (the medical conditions that prevent this are rare, but we still want to rule them out). You can then start to slowly decrease the supplementation and ensure that her weight continues to rise.

Your baby should still be feeding pretty often but not necessarily on a schedule yet. From an early age, some babies are grazers, preferring to feed every one and a half to two hours. Others are bingers and might already be spacing feedings out to nearly four hours. Your baby is still going to wake up a lot at night to feed. But *every* parent, including me, has had the experience of waking up in a panic after their baby's first six-hour stretch of sleep, wondering if she's okay. Did you ever think you'd feel guilty about getting six hours of sleep? Once she's up to her birth weight, though, trust that her body knows when and how much she needs to eat.

Your baby's job right now is to eat, sleep, poop, and be cute. I do ask if she looks toward your face or your voice occasionally, though. It is believed that babies at this age can see things less than two feet away and also probably contrasts, like something dark on a white wall. She can recognize your face, but she doesn't have much control of her eye muscles yet. So it's normal for her to cross her eyes or seem like she's looking past you.

SLEEP—A BITTERSWEET MEMORY

It's best not to dwell on it. Don't even think about those mornings when you would roll out of bed at nine after a fun night with friends, grab a latte, and then watch a little SportsCenter or HGTV to gather yourself. That never happened. You are on a different planet, in a different galaxy, in a different universe.

This is really about survival, about patching together as much sleep as possible and finding out what works best for your baby. Babies don't usually have any sort of schedule at this age. Over the first two weeks she's trying to get back to her birth weight, so she might wake every two hours to feed. Some babies are preset at birth to be more awake during the night and sleep more during the day. Don't panic if this is happening to you! This habit usually switches by about three weeks as she gets some hints from daytime light and your activity level.

The safest place for your baby to sleep at night is on her back in a bassinet, crib, co-sleeper, or play yard next to your bed. Yes, she'd rather be snuggled up next to you, and certainly cuddling with her while you're awake is a wonderful thing. However, it's quite clear that the risk of suffocation is higher when she's sleeping in bed with you (regardless of precautions you might take), so please think about that. Every parent I've talked to who co-sleeps says BUT. BUT I'm a light sleeper. BUT that's the only way she settles. BUT we have a king bed. It's true that co-sleeping is a part of many cultures. I'm sure that we did it for thousands of years, but we were probably more concerned about warmth and carnivores than SIDS (sudden infant death syndrome) at that time. The evidence regarding the risks of co-sleeping is too powerful to ignore. An extensive 2013 study[8] found that breastfeeding babies under three months old who share a bed with their parents are *five times* more likely to die from SIDS than those who sleep alone. You might still decide that co-sleeping works best for your family, but please consider that a crib or bassinet is safer for your child during her first year.

PROJECTILE VOMITING

Parents use the term pretty loosely, but real projectile vomiting is impressive (think *Poltergeist*). It literally can shoot a foot or two across the room! When this is constant or getting worse, it can be a sign of a rare condition called *pyloric stenosis*, where the next sphincter down the line (leading from the stomach to the intestines) is overgrown and blocks the milk from getting through. This needs to be checked out immediately, but a forceful burp in a happy baby is nothing to be concerned about.

Your baby should sleep on a firm mattress. She should *wear* most of what she needs to sleep with the exception of one thin blanket on top or swaddling her. Keep cute little comforters and stuffed animals out of the crib. And avoid the really comfy-looking padded crib bumpers, even if they do go perfectly with your nursery jungle theme. To a pediatrician, cute and comfy means suffocating. Mesh bumpers are safe and still prevent little arms and legs from poking out between slats.

Remember that at this age you can't spoil your baby. Nothing you do to make sleep better right now is setting up a bad habit (that comes later!), so try the swing, the swaddle (some babies love it and some hate it), the noise machine—whatever helps. And once she's crying, remember that she's still too young to soothe herself. So don't feel bad rushing in and picking her up. *But*, if she's just squirming and fussing a bit (again, babies can be quite snorty and grunty at night), it's fine to wait and see if she settles down.

THE SCOOP ON POOP

At two weeks, your baby should be pooping a *lot*, often after every single feed. She'll seem to take particular pleasure in pooping a little squirt, waiting for you to put on a fresh diaper, and then finishing up with a more impressive effort about thirty seconds later. Most poop at this age will be mustard yellow, seedy, and kind of watery. But anything that's yellow to green to orange to brown is fine. The only bad colors in the world of infant poop are red, black, and white. Pooping is your baby's biggest job, so don't be surprised if she grunts and gets red in the face for a few minutes while she's working it out.

A lot of parents get anxious when their baby's pooping slows down dramatically after one month. Some babies, particularly those who are breastfed, will suddenly go from pooping six times a day to pooping once every three or four days. Parents freak out because a twenty-fold difference in one week seems wrong. But the interval between poops doesn't really matter as long as she's feeding well. (A word of warning—the longer the interval, the more potential for a mega-blowout.)

Some babies do get constipated at this age, though. Be suspicious if she's straining and grunting for a long time but failing to pass anything. There are some safe ways of dealing with this. Giving her a warm bath really helps her intestines to relax (yes, I know this could create an Exxon Valdez–level disaster!). You can also use rectal stimulation, where you insert a metal-tip thermometer or petroleum jelly–covered cotton swab 1 centimeter into the anus and pull it out after twenty seconds. Surprisingly, this doesn't bother her and often triggers a pooping reflex that can provide some instant relief. If all else fails, you can use a bit of juice as medicine (this is about the *only* time that juice can help your child—see more on page 148): I recommend ½ to 1 ounce of apple or prune juice twice a day. You could give it via syringe or bottle and cut it with an equal amount of water if desired. If none of these methods seem to work, it's time to visit the doctor.

SPITTING UP (OR WHY YOU SHOULD MOTHBALL YOUR NICE CLOTHES FOR A WHILE)

Spitting up often gets worse after two weeks. Most babies do it at least once a day, but others will start to spit up after every single feeding. This can look like straight milk or like runny cottage cheese (a wonderful image) when it has already interacted with the stomach acid. It can be pretty forceful when an air bubble pushes it out. Spitting up is usually okay, as long as your baby is still happy and gaining great weight. But my gosh, sometimes it looks like the whole feeding came out! An ingenious 2013 study[9] found that we parents tend to drastically overestimate the volume of the urp.

Some babies who spit up a lot could have reflux (gastroesophageal reflux disease, or GERD). This is a condition where acid is often washing up and down your baby's esophagus (the tube leading from the mouth to the stomach), just like heartburn in adults. This usually happens because the sphincter valve between the esophagus and the stomach is not very tight yet. These babies are *fussy*. They spit up a lot but also are not very happy about it. Due to simple gravity, their symptoms are worse when lying down, so they often arch their backs and cry while they're lying back to sleep or feed. You can help by keeping your baby upright for at least fifteen minutes after feeding and slightly elevating the head of the crib with a few books or a rolled-up towel under the mattress. If she's still struggling, then it's time to see your pediatrician to discuss some other options. Spitting up and reflux often don't improve until after four to six months, when that sphincter muscle gets a little tighter and increasing amounts of solid foods are more likely to stay put in the stomach.

FUSSINESS AND ITS EVIL COUSIN, COLIC

Most babies start to cry more after two weeks, and not just when they're hungry or need to be changed. You've already handled that. But you might find that your baby also has a time during the late evening (7 p.m. to 11 p.m. or so—the "witching hour") where she's just kind of off. She might cry a lot even when fed and dry, and it might be hard to console her. This is normal and usually not too bad.

Some babies, though, maybe one in five, will cry a lot more and a lot harder. This may be *colic*. The official medical definition of colic is "when your baby cries all the time, and it's pretty awful, and you can't do anything to stop it, but she's still healthy and thriving." The "rule of threes" is a decent estimation of when fussiness crosses the line to become colic: three hours of crying per day, at least three days a week, for at least three straight weeks.

Medical professionals really don't understand colic very well. I think it's obvious to most parents that an unhappy tummy is at least a big part of it. Colicky babies grunt a lot and their tummies can feel like tight little drums. Their digestive system is still immature, and they can't move gas along quite as well as adults can. That trapped gas can stretch their little intestines, which is painful. They also have an immature nervous system, and that probably plays a role too. Babies are starting to be awake more after two weeks, and they're getting more stimulation. So sometimes their nerves can be a bit "fried" by the end of the day. And once they are crying hard, that immature nervous system can make it difficult to settle down again (just like when they get the hiccups and can't stop it).

Colic is *stressful*. Nature designed your baby's cry to electrify your emotions so you meet her needs. You feel a burst of adrenaline, a faster heart rate, and a higher blood pressure. This is a great way to be in a one-time survival situation, but it's really tough when it goes on for weeks at a time. When you're feeling like doing some inconsolable crying yourself, remember these two very important things:

1. Colic will never hurt your baby. If your baby is not developing appropriately or gaining good weight, something else is going on.

2. Colic ends, kind of magically, around three months.

Now let's talk about what you can do to make it better:

GOOD, AGGRESSIVE BURPING. It makes sense that the more air we can get out of that tummy, the happier your baby will be. Many parents I see burp their babies as if they're made of porcelain. But it's okay to pat just about as hard as you can while leaving the heel of your hand against your baby's back. Also, try breaking up a feed with several burps. Remember that your baby is probably gulping more air when she's frantic at the beginning of a feed than when she's winding down.

FINE TUNE YOUR BURPING STYLE

To keep her awake—Sit your baby up on your thigh facing away from you or to the side, then reach around and cup your hand gently around her neck and collarbone. Burp her with your other hand. You'll notice that her arms shoot out in front of her like she's casting a spell. This keeps her alert and works well when she's not done feeding yet, and you don't want her to fall asleep.

To get her to sleep—Curl her up, knees to chest with her face at your shoulder, and burp her with your opposite hand. That fetal position makes her want to sleep, so this is ideal when you're trying to get her down for a nap after feeding.

TUMMY COMFORT MEASURES. While lying back yourself, try placing your baby facedown on your chest with her knees drawn up to her chest. This is a comfy position that takes some pressure off her tummy and makes it easier to toot. You can also lay her on her back and gently bicycle her legs up and down. Heat, given with a bath or a warm washcloth over the tummy, is very soothing as well. You can also rub her tummy clockwise (the direction the colon moves in) while applying the heat. I think this stuff really does help—plus it gives you something to work on during a stressful time.

TAKE A BREAK. I can't overstate the importance of this for parents of colicky babies. When it's been thirty minutes and nothing you're doing is helping, it's OK to set your baby down in a safe place and walk to another room for a few minutes. (It's hard, but honestly, I'll bet you have no problem doing the same thing when your partner is fussy for only like five minutes.) Sometimes all that rocking, singing, and shushing can be a bit overstimulating for an immature nervous system. Also, friends and family want to help you—don't be afraid to ask! People love babies, especially when they get to turn them back in. Going out and having lunch with your partner or a friend can reenergize you. When you're stressed, your baby can sense it.

PROBIOTICS. This is good bacteria, the same stuff that's in yogurt. There is some evidence that babies with colic have an unhealthier balance of good bacteria in their intestines. Over the past few years, a handful of small studies suggested that giving probiotics might help. A 2017 meta-analysis[10] combined four of the best studies to strongly suggest that a particular probiotic (*Lactobacillus reuteri*) can reduce colic symptoms for breastfed babies. You can find the *L. reuteri* probiotics over the counter at your neighborhood pharmacy. Gerber sells them as "Soothe" probiotic colic drops.

Here are some things to be cautious about when trying to treat colic:

GAS DROPS (A.K.A. SIMETHICONE) AND GRIPE WATER. You've probably heard about these from friends. Lots of people use them. The problem is that no good evidence has ever shown that they're helpful. Gripe water is not regulated and can include a wide variety of undesirable ingredients such as alcohol. It has been linked to infections in the past as well.[11] I've never seen a baby get hurt from either of these, but I don't recommend them.

EXCESSIVE CHANGES IN YOUR DIET. As a breastfeeding mom, it's really important to eat a good varied diet. So try to avoid making big changes to figure out if something you're eating is making your baby fussy. Moms come into my clinic all the time saying they eat only boiled chicken and rice because they've taken dairy, soy, eggs, and wheat out of their diets. It's almost never the answer. Your baby *can* be sensitive to what you eat, but that is the exception (see page 59 for more on this in Milk Protein Intolerance). Your breast milk is a pretty good filter. Even though there's no direct evidence that gas-inducing foods you eat (like cabbage and beans) in turn make your baby gassier, many of my veteran moms would swear that they do. So moderating these foods is a reasonable thing you can do to try to help.

THE "FORMULA CAROUSEL." There are a lot of formulas out there, and many parents who formula feed are hopeful that the right one will end their baby's fussiness. I often meet parents who are switching rapidly from formula to formula when things don't improve after a few days. But babies can take a week to adjust to a new formula! Just know that in most cases a new formula is not the answer (see page 21 regarding a formula-swapping study). Most formula manufacturers offer a "gentle" product, where they break up the dairy proteins in the formula to theoretically make it easier to digest. There's no great evidence that this helps colic, but you could certainly try it. If you're at your wits' end, talk to your pediatrician, who might consider trying a special formula with proteins that are even more broken up.

A WORD ON BABY BLUES AND POSTPARTUM DEPRESSION

I know dads are dealing with some changes too, but they're nothing compared to what Mom is going through. Pregnancy and giving birth are exhausting, and right afterward hormones in your body plummet. When you add sleep deprivation and the anxiety of taking care of a newborn, your emotions can be overwhelming. This is why a majority of new moms get the "baby blues," a scientific term for feeling exhausted, unhappy, and worried at times after giving birth. These symptoms are usually mild and go away on their own within a couple of weeks. A lot of moms feel guilty and selfish about being unhappy after an event that's supposed to be so joyous. So I think it helps to know how common those feelings are. Follow your baby's cues, take care of yourself, and be honest about how you're feeling with the people you trust.

For some moms, however, these bad feelings get more intense and last longer. This can be a sign of postpartum depression, which affects more than 10 percent of new moms. The symptoms are basically the same as "regular" depression and usually start within a month of birth. Some of the most common are:

- Persistent feelings of sadness, worthlessness, or being inadequate as a new mom
- Changes in sleep—either oversleeping or having difficulty getting to sleep, and feeling extremely tired regardless of how much sleep you get
- Not being interested in the things you used to enjoy doing

- Withdrawing from friends and family and spending most of your time alone
- Change in appetite, whether it is eating more or less
- Frequent physical aches and pains, such as headache and sore muscles
- Not taking care of your own basic hygiene

The stakes are higher with postpartum depression because it affects how you bond and interact with your baby. Even if it only lasts for a few months, it can affect mother-baby interactions and therefore long-term development.[12] So know how common it is, and start by talking to *your* doctor if you think you might have it. Doctors are getting better at screening for postpartum depression, and partners should look out for it as well. Do *not* be afraid to ask for help from family or friends. Your health and your baby are too important for you to worry about imposing on someone.

MOMS' (OR DADS') GROUPS

Raising a baby will be one of the best experiences you'll ever have. But it can also be one of the loneliest. If your partner goes back to work, being alone at home with a baby can be very isolating—and it's okay to admit that. Throughout my career I've been amazed at the role moms' (or dads') groups play for parents. Some are impromptu, starting before the birth with labor or parenting classes, and others are longstanding groups in a particular community. They are places for you to socialize, exercise, get advice, give advice, and trade stuff. You won't be judged for breastfeeding there or for meltdowns (yours or your baby's!). And as your child gets older, she'll have a group of peers to play with. Above all you'll have support, which is crucial for keeping this whole thing afloat.

WAYS TO GIVE YOUR BABY A BOOST

Start giving your baby "tummy time." This means laying her on her tummy on a flat, firm surface (not just your chest) while awake. This strengthens her back, neck, and shoulders so that she gets better at moving. It also gets her off the back of her head, which will help it to stay round (flat heads are the scourge of back sleeping—see page 67 for more on this). Babies almost universally hate tummy time because they feel kind of helpless. So keep it brief—three minutes three times a day is a great start—and you can build from there.

Your baby's eyes are getting better every day. You can help this along by giving her things to track, or follow, with her eyes. Your face probably works best, but you can also use simple bright objects. When she's alert, just slowly move your head or the object in her field of view. It takes a lot of muscle control for her to keep her eyes on the prize, and by two months she'll be decent at it.

This is also a good time to start giving your baby some vitamin D, the one vitamin that's at very low levels in breast milk. The other usual sources are direct sunlight (no, it's not okay for your baby to tan quite yet) and fortified milk (which shouldn't be offered until twelve months). Vitamin D is really important for forming strong bones, among other things. It's available in two forms for babies: a liquid given 1 milliliter at a time with a medicine dropper and a more concentrated "drop" form. I love the drops because they are just mixed in coconut oil without any dyes, and you can put the drop right at the breast. Plan on giving vitamin D daily as long as you breastfeed.

A final word for the two-week mark: Just enjoy your baby. Notice how she reacts differently to you than to other people, how she looks toward *your* face and turns toward *your* voice. Be proud that you know how to give her everything she needs already. Think about how she'll sound when she eventually talks, how she'll look when she's five, and what sports she might play. Think about what you want her to eat, the role you want screens to play in her life, what kind of manners you want to teach her. We all want our kids to be better than ourselves, and that takes thoughtful planning. Have fun considering all the possibilities.

FAQS

My baby has this weird red rash with little yellow welts in the middle. Is it hives? Lupus?

It's probably not lupus (isn't it annoying that doctors will never say anything is 100 percent?). This is a really common newborn rash that about half of babies get to some degree. It has one of the all-time worst names for a benign condition—*erythema toxicum.* That sounds like some kind of medieval plague, but it's completely innocent. You'll notice that the rash moves around on your baby's skin throughout the day, but it doesn't bother her and usually resolves by about three weeks. No need to get this one evaluated.

My baby sneezes and gets the hiccups a lot. Is that normal? Is she allergic to something?

These are really the two things that *all* babies do until two to three months. Sneezing at this age is never caused by an allergy—environmental allergies usually take a few years to develop. It's actually kind of a useful reflex to keep the nose clear and eliminate infections that might be settling there. The hiccups are just annoying—they're caused by spasming of the diaphragm, a thin sheet of muscle between the stomach and the lungs that gets worked pretty hard at this age. Hiccups will always resolve on their own, but sometimes giving a pacifier or something from a dropper (like vitamin D) stops them.

We're getting cabin fever—can we take our baby out anywhere before two months?

Absolutely! I think this is important for both you and your baby. Your baby is not as fragile as she seems right now. Mom, for the next few months she's got good antibodies from your blood that help protect her from everything you've ever been exposed to. Plus, the antibodies in breast milk add another layer of protection. Finally, remember that kids don't usually get sick because another kid coughs on them. They get sick from *surfaces*—touching something that another snotty kid touched an hour ago. And newborns aren't doing that yet.

Go on as many walks as you can, even in winter. She'll be warm enough. I'm always fascinated at how being outside seems to calm babies—maybe it's the breeze or just getting some more visual input. Don't hesitate at all to take your baby to places that are fairly open, such as a grocery store or a spacious restaurant. Newborns usually do great on two- to three-hour car trips as well. She'll probably sleep most of the way except for a few feeding stops.

I think it's reasonable to try to avoid places that are closed in and a bit denser, like a church nursery or an airplane. A higher concentration of people means a higher concentration of germs. Family gatherings are fine—just beware of toddlers who are still learning how to control their secretions.

OK, it seems like for any weird thing we bring up, you tell us it's normal. So please tell me it's normal that my infant son is growing breasts.

It's normal. (Probably half of what I do at the two-week visit is tell people that stuff is normal.) The same hormones that increase a mother's breast size and milk supply leading up to birth also affect girl *and* boy babies. These hard lumps of real breast tissue under the nipples can get bigger over the first few weeks. Milk can even come out of the nipple! There's nothing you need to do—the tissue will slowly shrink over the next few months. Like any breast tissue, it can occasionally get infected, so see your pediatrician if the area gets red and warm.

What about everything I had to avoid when I was pregnant, like coffee and alcohol and seafood? I've been thinking about that stuff lately . . .

Fortunately, food restrictions loosen up a bit now. Developing fetal brains are incredibly sensitive to little insults. Breast milk is a pretty good filter, though, and it's harder for things to get from your blood to her blood now. So some coffee is okay, but I'd max out at one strong cup a day. More than that and your baby may get a bit jittery. There's still a slight concern with mercury, so just be reasonable with the amount of "top ocean predators" you eat (tuna, shark, mackerel—does anyone eat mackerel?). You still have to be careful with alcohol. It's eliminated at a constant rate from both your blood and your breast milk. A good limit for a 150-pound mother is 8 ounces of wine, two beers, or 2 ounces of liquor on occasion, and you should wait three to four hours to breastfeed again. "Pump and dump" doesn't speed this along and is really only helpful if you're getting engorged before it's safe to nurse again.

Vaccines!

I just took three big breaths—in through my nose, out through my mouth—and I suggest you do the same. Vaccines are a hot-button issue. I briefly fantasized that I could write a parenting book without addressing them, but they're just too important. So we'll keep it relaxed, and I'll talk to you about vaccines like I talk to my patients.

When I started as a pediatrician, vaccines *lit my fire*. I would come at parents with a mountain of beautiful data and studies that would crush all the misperceptions they had about vaccines. They would then politely decline all of the immunizations, and we'd have some lingering awkwardness. A 2014 study[13] basically confirmed that a heavy-handed strategy isn't a very effective one—emphasizing how severe the illnesses are or how safe the vaccines are actually *decreased* parents' intentions to vaccinate! This tells me that vaccines are an emotional issue rather than a scientific one for many parents. When people feel attacked or cornered on an emotional issue, they get defensive and dig in. That's human nature.

So any discussion about vaccines has to start with respect. You are trying to make the best decisions for your kid, and your doctor is trying to keep your kid as healthy as possible. I try to make my respect for parents clear with my number one rule: *You have to be comfortable with the choice you make for your kid.*

First, here's a quick rundown on the vaccines your child needs at two, four, and six months. These are grouped into two or three injections, with another given by mouth. A lot of the facts I use in this section are from the CDC, and their Vaccine Information Statement website is an excellent place to learn more.[14]

A COMMUNITY-BASED MODEL FOR INCREASING VACCINATION RATES

It's easy to get pessimistic about declining vaccination rates, especially when evidence suggests that counseling from doctors alone is not very helpful. So what can we do? Boost Oregon is an exciting organization in my state that is taking a novel approach to the problem. Nadine Gartner, a mom and non-medical professional, founded the organization in 2015. It's a grassroots effort consisting of parents, doctors, nurses, naturopaths, midwives, and others with the common goal of sharing accurate information about vaccines. Anti-vaccine beliefs spread through communities of parents who trust each other and have emotional connections, and Boost Oregon believes that it takes a similar community-based effort to change those beliefs. "Vaccine-hesitant parents are fearful because of misinformation that they have read online or heard from their loved ones," notes Gartner, "and they likely absorbed that misinformation over a period of months or even years. No matter how skilled the medical provider, that hesitancy will not dissipate in a single well-check visit."

The organization uses both private and public funding (but *not* pharmaceutical money) to run free community workshops for new and expecting parents, train medical professionals and parent volunteers on how to effectively talk about vaccines, and distribute non-judgemental pamphlets that help parents work through the facts and myths of vaccines. I think it's a promising model for helping new parents be comfortable with vaccines. Check it out at BoostOregon.org.

DTAP. This and the pneumococcal vaccine are the biggies for most doctors. It does prevent diphtheria, which can affect your breathing and heart, and tetanus, which you get from a dirty cut and can lead to muscle spasms (particularly in the jaw). Most importantly for babies, however, it protects them from pertussis, also known as whooping cough. For adults, pertussis is a really awful intense cough that can last for twelve weeks. But it can cause infants to stop breathing and fill their blood with so many white blood cells that it gets sludgy. And we haven't found a good way to keep adults vaccinated long-term, so there are a lot of potential exposures. It takes kids five doses of DTaP by kindergarten to be up to date, but even the first one offers significant protection against pertussis. DTaP is a bit more likely than some of the other vaccines to cause a day or two of fever, but your baby can handle that.

PNEUMOCOCCAL. This vaccine protects against thirteen strains of bacteria that cause "pneumococcal disease." These are severe diseases such as pneumonia, meningitis, and blood infections. The CDC reports that the vaccine has cut serious incidents due to these illnesses by 88 percent in kids under age five. That's massive. The vaccine has helped to reduce the rate of ear infections as well, which is not a huge deal until your kid is screaming with one in the middle of the night. Your child will usually get four of these vaccines by twelve months.

HIB. This vaccine protects against a bacteria called *Haemophilus influenzae type b*. This used to be a devastating illness that was the top cause of bacterial meningitis in kids younger than five. About 20,000 kids got it each year in the United States and around 5 percent of them died. The vaccine has cut these infections by an astonishing *99 percent* since it came out just over thirty years ago. That's one of the biggest success stories for kids' health over the past fifty years. Guess how many cases I've seen in my career? Zero. Guess how many severe side effects I've seen from *thousands* of doses of the vaccine? Zero. Babies will get three or four of these vaccines by twelve months.

ROTAVIRUS. Rotavirus causes *bad* diarrhea in children under five. Prior to the introduction of the vaccine in 2006, it was easily the biggest cause of severe diarrhea in children under five.[15] About 400,000 children in the United States had to go to the doctor each year for rotavirus and nearly 70,000 had to be hospitalized. The vaccine has made severe rotavirus infections rare today. It's also nice that it's given by mouth, with mild vomiting or diarrhea being a rare side effect. Since it's a live vaccine, talk to your doctor if your baby has serious problems with his immune system. It's the only vaccine with some time restrictions. Your child has to get his first dose by fifteen weeks and the last dose by eight months. There will be a total of two or three depending on which form he is given.

HEPATITIS B. This virus can cause an acute illness with fever, fatigue, jaundice, and muscle pain. The real danger, however, is that 90 percent of the infants who contract Hep B develop a long-term infection that damages their liver (up to one in four will die from liver complications). Babies most often get the virus from infected moms during birth—most moms are tested for it but the test is imperfect. Babies can get Hep B from other caregivers too. This is why we usually start the vaccine at birth. Hep B can be spread later through any body fluid, and fortunately the protection from the vaccine is lifelong. This vaccine has fewer side effects than other vaccines and is given in a series of three shots over the first six months of life.

IPV (POLIO). Here is another phenomenal success story that we've lost all perspective on. Thousands of people were paralyzed or killed *each year* by polio virus before the vaccine came out in 1955. There are still a lot of older Americans alive today with disabilities due to childhood polio infections. Because of the vaccine, *it has been completely eradicated in the United States*. That's remarkable. But it still exists in some parts of the world, and it would only take one infected traveler to bring it back here. If everyone keeps getting vaccinated, we have an excellent chance of eliminating polio forever in the next few decades (just like smallpox). Then no more vaccine would be needed! Your child gets three shots over the first six months and one more before kindergarten.

The media tends to portray vaccines as a controversial issue. They interview a pro-vaccine person, then an anti-vaccine person. There are a dizzying number of articles, blogs, and social media postings all over the internet about both opinions. So I think many parents perceive that, even in the medical community, there is a lot of controversy. They even ask me what I think about vaccines and if I would get them for my children. I want to tell you that in the pediatrics community there is virtually *no* controversy over vaccines. We all love them and we all get our kids vaccinated as soon as possible. We think they are probably the single most important thing we do for our patients. We don't have the *opinion* that vaccines make kids healthier—we *know* they do. We have also seen the kids who suffer when they get one of the diseases a vaccine could have prevented. We have tons of opinions about other stuff, but this is a simple fact for us. We're parents *and* scientists, so we know how to evaluate sixty years of evidence. That may not sway your decision, but it's important to acknowledge.

Let's address a few common concerns about vaccines:

1. **IT'S TOO HARD ON MY BABY'S BODY TO GET THAT MANY VACCINES AT ONCE.** The recommended vaccine schedule is pretty busy the first year, to be sure. This causes some parents to want to space out the vaccines. But your child is most vulnerable to these serious diseases during the first year, so we're kind of in a rush to protect him. Your baby has an extensive, powerful immune system—remember that each vaccine is just revving up a small part of it. An older study from 1994[16] looked at the stress caused by vaccines as measured by infants' cortisol. Cortisol is a chemical produced by our bodies in response to stress, and infants seem to have

similar cortisol increases whether they receive one or two vaccines at the same time. Splitting up the vaccines simply creates more stressful interactions.

Also, when you come back to get more vaccines a month after they are due (such as by following Dr. Bob's alternative vaccine schedule—see page 54), your child is less protected at any one point in time. Bottom line, if a spaced-out schedule is what it takes for you to vaccinate your child, do it. But please consider that the recommended schedule exists for a reason.

2. THERE ARE SO MANY MORE VACCINES TODAY THAN WHEN WE WERE KIDS. There are several more, yes, but it's all about the antigens, baby! (Bumper sticker?) Antigens are the little pieces in the vaccine (mostly proteins) your immune system forms a response to. It's the number of antigens rather than the number of vaccines that determines how hard your child's immune system has to work after getting them. And the number of vaccine antigens a child is exposed to by age two has been reduced *drastically*, from about 3,000 in 1980 to about 150 today.[17] Vaccines have simply become more streamlined and more efficient. So your kiddo is not only better protected than you were, he has less stress on his immune system to boot.

3. I'M CONCERNED ABOUT ALL THE CRAP IN VACCINES. Here is a true statement: there is mercury, aluminum, and formaldehyde in vaccines. That stuff is all toxic! But it's *everywhere*, and it's all about *amounts*. A 2003 paper by Paul Offit and Rita Jew does a wonderful job of addressing this issue[18] (it's written in language that interested parents can understand). Aluminum is an *adjuvant*, which helps to carry the parts of the vaccine your immune system responds to. Offit and Jew point out that your baby will get more aluminum from breast milk or formula than vaccines.

Mercury is also in everything we eat to some degree. Thimerosal is a mercury-containing compound that was used as a preservative in several vaccines to prevent bacteria and fungus from growing. Thimerosal was taken out of most childhood vaccines in 2001. A 2002 study looked at mercury levels of six-month-olds who had received the routine thimerosal-containing vaccines and found they were within recommendations.[19] Even though the older vaccines were safe, vaccines today have far less mercury because they are usually given from "single dose" vials that don't need as much preservative.

Finally, formaldehyde is used to kill or inactivate the viruses in some vaccines (your body can still recognize these dead viruses and form a nice response to them), so a little bit ends up in the vaccine. No vaccine has more than 0.1 milligram. Offit and Jew point out that the average two-month-old has 1.1 milligrams in her blood anyway, because it's needed for certain chemical pathways in our bodies.

4. **MY NIECE AND NEPHEW HAVE NEVER HAD VACCINES, AND THEY ARE AS HEALTHY AS CAN BE.** It's very true that if you live in a community where most people vaccinate, your child has a great chance of staying healthy even without vaccines. *Only* because everyone else is vaccinated. That's called *herd immunity*, where enough people are vaccinated that outbreaks have a hard time getting going. But it's so fragile! When the percentage of vaccinated people falls below about 90 percent (a bit more or less depending on the disease), herd immunity crumbles. As vaccination rates have fallen in certain areas, we have seen new outbreaks of diseases that were previously nearly eliminated in the United States, including a well-publicized measles outbreak at Disneyland in 2015 and a nationwide mumps outbreak in 2017.

> I know that you are making this decision for *your* child, not for the community, and I respect that distinction. But understand that there are children with fragile immune systems who can't get vaccines. They depend on herd immunity. And be aware that even if most others are vaccinated (and you probably won't know exactly what percentage are), these diseases are still a real risk to your child.

A small but growing number of pediatricians have decided to no longer see patients who don't follow the recommended vaccine schedule. I understand their reasoning. Many parents who do vaccinate or have children with poor immune systems like this policy as well. But I don't. Yes, you don't want your kid catching measles from another kid in the waiting room, but these people are also part of your community. I would rather develop a relationship with them, earn their trust, and work toward a reasonable vaccine plan than have them go to another clinic where that might not happen.

I hope you ultimately decide to get all the recommended vaccines for your child. I hope you trust your pediatrician and value her opinion on the issue above that of a celebrity or a Facebook friend. I hope you feel that you can raise concerns and ask questions about vaccines without being judged. And most of all, I hope you feel good about whatever choices you make for your family.

DR. BOB'S ALTERNATIVE VACCINE SCHEDULE

Dr. Robert Sears is a pediatrician who has written several books. In 2007 he published *The Vaccine Book: Making the Right Decision for Your Child*. This was a time when there was a lot of anxiety over vaccines. Dr. Bob does not say vaccines are bad, and to be fair, he refers to himself as pro-vaccine. But he devotes much of the book to validating that anxiety and raising concerns (without many conclusions) about additives in vaccines, side effects, pharmaceutical company shadiness, and even how big of a problem the diseases really are. After creating an atmosphere of anxiety, he swoops in with an alternative vaccine schedule to save the day.

The schedule involves delaying some vaccines such as MMR and hepatitis B, and spacing out the others so that no more than two vaccines are ever given at a time. This requires nineteen vaccine visits to the doctor before kindergarten rather than seven with the recommended schedule. I'm not sure your baby would appreciate that! It's also important to remember that this alternative vaccine schedule is based on *absolutely nothing*. Dr. Sears took the anxiety that many parents have about vaccines, reinforced it with his MD credentials, and then made up a solution. He would say that the alternative schedule gets some parents to vaccinate who otherwise might not. That may be true. But parents who follow Dr. Bob's vaccine schedule are still leaving their babies more vulnerable to serious diseases with no science to back it up.

Two Months

Things are starting to get exciting. Day and night might still be blurred into a delirium of diapers, feeding, and spit-up, but all your hard work is paying off. Your baby is starting to be awake for longer chunks of time. She's starting to do more than eat, poop, grunt, and sleep. She's developing a little personality and beginning to interact with you and the world around her. More time awake means that she's ready to learn, and you are the only teachers she really cares about. It's exciting to be the teacher, but that daunting responsibility can cause a lot of anxiety for new parents as well. Let's get to it.

WHAT YOUR BABY SHOULD BE DOING NOW

Most importantly, your baby should be growing well—this includes height, weight, and head circumference. Pediatricians use percentiles to keep track of these metrics, and yours will usually show you the growth chart. If your baby's weight is at the 70th percentile, that means if you took one hundred random girls her age, she'd weigh more than seventy of them and less than about thirty of them. Realize that your baby might move around the growth chart quite a bit during the first twelve months. As long as the weight and height are moving around together, then there's nothing to worry about.

Babies come in all shapes and sizes just like adults. If a baby is always around the 80th percentile for height and the 30th percentile for weight, that's perfectly normal. She's a long, skinny baby. But if I see a baby who is at the 80th percentile for height and her weight has fallen from the 80th to the 40th percentile over several months, that could be a problem. Growth is really important and kind of complicated. Don't hesitate to ask your doctor to show you your child's growth chart and help you get comfortable with it.

BIG OLD BABY HEADS

These problems are rare, but if your baby's head is growing too fast, we become concerned about something called *hydrocephalus*. This means "water on the brain." Our bodies are constantly making new fluid that bathes the brain and spinal cord. If the "drains" that get rid of the old fluid get clogged, all that extra pressure expands the skull (which is soft and flexible for months after birth). Lots of kids have massive heads that are stable on the growth chart—and I can usually glance at their parents' sizable noggins and see why! On the other hand, if your baby's head circumference is not consistently increasing, that may mean her brain is not growing enough. Most pediatricians check head measurements until two years old.

Your baby's vision should be getting pretty sharp. She should be able to look at you across a small room and focus on your eyes, and she should be able to smoothly move her eyes to follow you. This is called tracking. Of course, she might stare at a fan for ten minutes too, so don't expect to see this all the time.

Your baby should be doing some cooing. This means making some oohs and aahs rather than just the gassy grunts you've gotten used to. Realize that some babies are chatterboxes and make sounds almost constantly (good luck when she's three!), while others are a bit more observant and might only talk a few times a day. Both are great.

Perhaps the sweetest thing your baby should start doing around now is smiling. Not just the milk-drunk dreaming smile she's done since birth, but a smile back at you when you smile at her. We call this a "social smile," and it shows that she understands a smile is something special. It's also the first sign that she's getting obsessed with you.

Finally, from all her little tummy time exercises, she should be able to lift her head off the ground a bit, maybe to forty-five degrees, and look around a few times before it plops back down. She still doesn't realize that her arms are attached to her body, but she'll likely bat at things and clench anything her fingers come across. It's just more of an accident at two months.

PATIENCE WITH PREEMIES

We consider babies born before thirty-seven weeks to be premature. It's important to realize that these babies are on their own special tracks for growth and development. We use their "full-term" age when considering both. So, for a girl born at 35 weeks who is now two months old, we would plot her on the growth chart as a one-month-old. We would expect her to hit her "two-month milestones" around three months. If she does some things earlier, fantastic—but be patient! She'll get there, and she's likely to catch up on size and development by one to two years. Your pediatrician may want to see your preemie a bit more often than the regular well-check schedule just to make sure she's closing the gap.

MY BABY IS STILL FUSSY!

Six to eight weeks is probably the peak of colic. So if your baby is still feeding well, meeting milestones, and growing well at the two-month appointment, it's likely that. But the end is in sight—remember that colic usually goes away around three months. Also, keep in mind that reflux could still be worsening at this age. If she's arching and seems uncomfortable while lying down or during feeds, call your doctor.

QUICK FEEDING UPDATE

You and your baby should be in a pretty good rhythm by now. A lot of parents ask, "How much and how often should my baby be feeding?" The answer is, "As much and as often as she needs to gain good weight." Seriously, it's all over the map. The average might be 4 ounces every three hours at two months. But some babies are grazers who take 2.5 ounces every two hours, and others are bingers who pound 6 ounces every four hours. The bottom line is that your baby knows what she needs, so follow her cues! And don't even think about solids yet—that's a conversation to start with your pediatrician at four months.

One problem that comes up for many nursing moms heading back to work is the "bottle strike." You've worked hard to fill your freezer with pumped milk for bottle feeding when you're gone. But she's not into it! She might take only 3 or 4 ounces over the entire day! And the five types of bottles you've bought don't help. You don't need me to tell you this is stressful, especially when you're already sad to be away from your little one for so long. But let me give you some reassurance! Even when she's just scraping by during the day, she'll load up at the breast in the morning and when you get home. Her drive to get the calories she needs is super strong. I have *never* seen a bottle strike affect

MILK PROTEIN INTOLERANCE

This is a somewhat common (maybe 5 to 10 percent of infants) condition in which a baby's intestines get irritated from dairy products. The culprit is usually dairy in Mom's diet that finds its way into the breast milk, or cow-milk proteins in typical formula. It is different from a true *allergy,* which often causes hives and vomiting. The symptoms can overlap with both colic and reflux, so I think it's important to recognize the differences. These kids are fussy too, but not more during the evening as in colic or more when lying down as with reflux. They tend to spit up a lot and they can be rashy. Colic is easing up as babies approach three months, but milk protein intolerance is often getting worse at that time. The clincher is when there is some blood in her stool, which happens about 50 percent of the time in babies with milk protein intolerance.

This condition is easy to treat for formula-fed babies by switching to special formulas with chopped-up dairy proteins. It's tougher for breastfeeding moms, because we usually try cutting dairy out of their diet to see if things improve. Fortunately, some newer research suggests that it resolves in most kids by seven to ten months.[20] About one-fourth of affected infants will also have trouble with soy, so your doctor might have you cut that out of your diet as well.

a baby's growth. So try to relax, and tell whoever is doing the bottle feeding to do the same. Trying to force feedings on a baby who doesn't want them can go to a bad place. (Was it still stressful when my own son did this? You bet.)

What about water? Your baby doesn't really need it—she gets all the hydration she needs from breast milk or formula. However, a small amount can be okay if your baby is older than two months. One example might be if you're out somewhere on a hot summer day and in between feeds. A good rule of thumb is that your baby could safely have as many ounces of water in a twenty-four-hour period as she is months old. So a two-month-old could safely have 2 ounces of water and a four-month-old could safely have 4 ounces. Your baby's immature kidneys would have a hard time peeing out any more than this, which could cause her blood to become too diluted, so don't go overboard.

SETTING YOURSELF UP FOR SLEEP SUCCESS

You are now a grizzled veteran of sleep deprivation. You can function on levels of sleep used to weed out soldiers during Special Forces training. But you also have a friend whose two-month-old is sleeping through the night. Even if she's nice about it, you'll have to get rid of this friend—it's just not going to work out. And while hope can be a dangerous thing, there is light at the end of the tunnel.

Between two and four months is a big transition time for sleep. Your baby still can't soothe herself very well, but she's going to get better at it over the next two months. There are some things we can do now to *set up* good sleep for your baby. If you have a separate room and crib, this next month is a good time to think about getting her in there. When she's right next to you, she sees and smells you every time she's half-awake, so she's more likely to fully awaken and look for some soothing. But if she's in her own space she has a few things she can start to work on, like shifting around and sucking her hands. If putting her in another room makes you nervous, remember that you still have your monitor and will probably pop awake every time she scratches her nose.

You can also start to put her to bed when she's drowsy, but not conked out, after a feeding. Yes, she'll probably startle awake most of the time. And once she's full-out crying, you're done—you should still comfort her right away because she can't quite settle down from that yet. *But* if she's just grunting, squirming, or fussing a bit, give her some time to work it out before intervening. You'll get fidgety, so try to hum a little song to yourself for a couple minutes and see if she's relaxed by the time you finish.

You know that reflex where your baby gets startled and throws her hands out to the sides, waking herself up? The one that looks like the earth is shaking beneath her? Well, that goes away by three months. So you don't really need the swaddle to prevent it anymore. Three months is a good time to start taking away the swaddle and other things, such as swings and white noise, that were crucial for the first few months but can become crutches that hinder self-soothing by four months.

Before two months, most babies really don't have much of a napping "schedule." In fact, naps can be kind of a disaster—napping for fifteen minutes in the car, then being up for five hours, napping for twenty-five minutes in the stroller, popping awake during the transfer to the crib, and so on. While a set schedule is still a fantasy at two to three months, there is a simple technique you can use to at least shape her naps up. When your baby wakes up, *regardless of how long she's been sleeping*, a ninety-minute clock starts ticking. At the end of that ninety minutes, your baby's brain is ready to sleep again. If you miss that window, then her brain has moved on and you're likely in for a shorter nap or an even longer awake period. I know it seems a bit anal to record the time that your baby wakes up, but it works! Especially for babies under four months old. The result is longer naps that allow you to get some other things done and a happier baby to play with when she wakes up.

TOXIC STRESS

We've known for a long time that what happens to your baby—good and bad—can have long-lasting effects on her well-being. Not surprising. But recently researchers have focused on stress and the ripple effect it can have on developing brains.

Cortisol can be thought of as a stress hormone. When humans are stressed, whether through fear, anger, pain, or illness, our bodies pour cortisol into our blood. This makes us more alert, speeds up our hearts, and gets muscles ready to move (think of how you'd feel if a grizzly bear stepped onto the trail fifty feet ahead of you). This is an amazing response that lets you run away from lions and lift cars off people and stuff. But those are pretty rare occasions.

Now we know that your baby can have the same response to stress in her environment. When you and your spouse argue, she's stressed by the volume of your voice and your body language. If you are sad or depressed, she's stressed by getting less eye contact and fewer touches. This can put her body in a constant state of "fight or flight." Her little cortisol system can become twitchy and go a bit haywire, and these changes can become permanent. Those poor kids have difficulty regulating their emotions and coping with stress. They struggle with attention and relationships. They are less healthy and do more poorly in school or at almost anything else you can measure.[21]

I know this is some pretty heavy stuff, but a big focus in pediatrics right now is identifying toxic stress and trying to build resiliency against it. Awareness is the first step, and that's why I'm telling you about it. Just know that your baby is always watching to make sure her surroundings are safe and stable.

BUILDING A BRAIN

What's going to make your baby smarter—Beethoven or Bach? Trick question—it's Mozart. Just kidding. This is a really big point. Remember, all your baby cares about is your voice and your face. Everything you do—your words, your tone, your touch, your expressions—has a portal directly into her brain. These things you do and say don't just make her smile, they create lasting connections in her brain that will affect *everything*: her speech, her self-esteem, her ability to process emotions, and probably a lot of other capacities we don't realize yet. This might seem like a lot of pressure, but I think it's a tremendous opportunity for you. Unlike with other things in our society, you're not at a disadvantage if you have less money or education. You and your baby could spend the next year in a white room with a bare floor and bare walls, and she would have everything she needs for optimal brain development. This should empower you!

It's good to get in the habit of talking *constantly* to your baby. You could read her last night's sports scores. You could tell her about some awkward junior high moments. You could catch her up on the latest celebrity gossip. It doesn't matter. I encourage parents to just kind of narrate the day to their baby. Here's an example if you were walking outside: "There's a tree! See the tree? It's so big! The bark is rough—see how rough it feels? And so many leaves! See all the leaves? The leaves are green and they feel smooth—see how smooth they are?" Lots of repetition, simple descriptive words, and pretty much everything ends in an exclamation point or question mark.

You know that singsongy, high-pitched, dripping-with-inflection voice that used to annoy you before you had kids? Some call it "parentese." Well, there's good evidence to show that babies love that type of talk. They tend to turn their heads toward it more than regular adult tones—even when it's in a different language! As they get a bit older, they're more likely to respond to directions in parentese as well. This probably explains why all cultures, from hunter-gatherers to trendy Europeans, talk to their babies that way. Note that this is different from "baby talk," where you say nonsense words and partial syllables. Parentese uses regular words but with tons of inflection and drawn-out vowels.

One of my favorite studies followed children from three months to three years and kept track of how many words they heard from their caregivers.[22] The researchers found that children in families of higher socioeconomic status heard a mind-blowing thirty million more words throughout childhood than children living in poverty. They then found that the number of words was predictive of later success in school. It's sad that there's such variation in the number of words kids hear before heading into kindergarten, and that those gaps already put them on a track for success or failure. But it's also *hopeful*! We spend a lot of time talking about how to give kids a better life, and those discussions often focus on solutions that cost a lot of money. But anyone can talk! Empowering parents to talk a certain way to their kids can have a huge impact on children's development and their future.

You're also going to have to decide on the role you want screens and technology to play for your child, and the time to start thinking about that is now. Not many people are plopping their two-month-olds in front of a Disney movie yet. But a lot of people keep their TV on in the background all day long. Parents come in and tell me, "It's funny—he just loves the TV and turns his head to look at it!" Of course he likes it—it's bright and loud with rapidly changing images. But it's precisely that stimulation that's the problem for a developing brain (see page 168 for more on this). Also, remember that it's all about you right now, and screens or anything else that distracts your baby means less time learning from your face and words. Of course, I believe important sporting events are exempt from this concern and probably important for character development. (My wife disagrees . . .)

One study[23] out of the University of Washington on the effects of "educational" baby videos was rather shocking. The researchers found that watching such videos under the age of two actually resulted in kids learning fewer vocabulary words and performing worse on language skill tests! I think many of us expected that such videos didn't help babies, but the suggestion that they could actually *hurt* brain development was eye-opening.

Personally, my wife and I decided to move our only TV to the basement before our kids were born. Now we have to consciously go downstairs to watch it rather than having it on in the background or "checking the scores" throughout the day. This has worked great for us, and the kids just don't really think about it. This approach might not be right for your family, but I would encourage you to create some kind of concrete plan. If you tend to keep the TV on for background noise, for example, try music as a more brain-friendly way of accomplishing the same thing.

And then there are smartphones. Indispensable for most people. They let you instantly share pictures of your baby with your entire family. You can catch all of her milestones on video without having to warm up the camcorder. You can talk with Grandma and see her face when she's 3,000 miles away. But I worry about smartphones every day. The technology has advanced more quickly than our understanding of how it affects our brains and our relationships. I worry when I see a mom at the park, absent-mindedly pushing her quiet one-year-old in a swing while staring at her phone. I worry that it's perfectly acceptable to interact with your phone while sitting with a friend or family member at a restaurant. I worry when a dad's attention is divided between me and his phone while we're talking about his six-month-old in the office (what does he do when he's at home?).

Your kid is going to be really good at using a smartphone. You'll probably find some learning apps that teach her a few things, and it will be a crucial distraction for surviving long flights or car rides. But it will *never*, at any age, be a substitute for looking at your face and talking to you. When you are looking at your phone for a few minutes, that's a few facial expressions your baby's not learning from, and a few hundred words she's not hearing from you. So try to think about it ahead of time, realize how addictive it is, and aim to limit phone use when you're with your baby.

DISCLAIMER: I know I'm crusty about this stuff. A friend made a really good point that I should probably just call them "phones" now rather than "smartphones." Probably true, but "smartphone" distinguishes it from what I have, which is a "flip phone." It has big buttons for people with arthritis and a large cataract-friendly display. This whole "texting" fad is annoying because it takes me a long time to scroll through all the letters and reply. But when I'm with my kids, I'm *really* with my kids.

WAYS TO GIVE YOUR BABY A BOOST

Your baby wants to get strong over the next few months. You can help her by increasing the tummy time. If she still doesn't love it (a pretty safe bet), tolerate a little more fussing. You're probably not that happy during your workouts either! Remember, the more time she spends on her tummy (while awake), the less flat her head will be in the long run.

Another thing you can try is putting your hands under her armpits and lifting her up and down. This does two things—she'll brace against your hands to strengthen her shoulder area, and her eyes will have to work to focus on you as you move closer and farther away.

Most babies are just starting to put some weight on their legs at two months. Notice how she naturally wants to bounce. There's a myth out there that babies can get bow-legged if they spend too much time on their legs. Not at all true. I say it boosts her chances of becoming a powerlifter or a pro soccer player. Seriously though, if she gets tired of standing, she'll let you know it. Finally, notice how she'll push against your hands as you push her legs up toward her chest. That's another way to work on those thighs.

FAQS

I have to go back to work soon. Will daycare ruin my baby?

No. Be confident in the bond you have with your baby and the time you do get to spend with her. You're making the best choice you can to give her a solid future. As she gets older, daycare can be a pretty stimulating place. My best advice is to get a daycare referral from someone you trust. Interacting with a consistent caregiver gives your baby some of the same advantages we've talked about earlier in this chapter. And you can always drop in on your little one during your lunch break!

Our baby's head is kind of flat. Does she need a helmet? What can we do to fix it?

The "Back to Sleep" campaign has been one of the more successful public health efforts of the past twenty-five years, cutting the rate of SIDS nearly in half. The downside of having all those babies sleep on their backs is that we have a lot of flat heads now. It's purely cosmetic and doesn't affect brain development. The fancy word for this is *plagiocephaly*, and about half of babies have it to some degree by two months. Most of the time it's pretty random since some kids' skulls are softer than others. It's more common in preemies, babies who spend too much time on their backs, and babies who don't move their heads as much when they sleep. The flatness can be symmetric, or it can be more on one side versus the other.

Sometimes, flatness on one side of your baby's head can be a sign of a condition called *torticollis*. This happens when the muscles on one side of her neck are too tight, causing her to look one way more than the other. These babies tend to tilt their heads to one side as well. This condition can be helped by physical therapy and home exercises. More often than not, your baby might just *prefer* to look one way. You can help by turning her bassinet or crib so that she has to look the other way to see you. When you play with her, arrange it so that the rounded (not flat) side of her head is on the ground.

THE TORTLE

There's a simple, cheap, and ingenious product that can sometimes help with heads that are more flat on one side than the other. It's called the Tortle. It's a stylish little hat that has a soft foam roll on the back of it. You put it on your baby at night and put the foam roll over the flat area. It's a gentle way to have her sleep on the other side of her head. Unless she rips it off, which some babies do. You can buy it online or at Target.

Even though the flatness won't go away entirely using these methods, it's almost always okay. In my experience it usually does not get worse after four months. After that your baby's head will start to get a bit rounder, and she will get more hair. Everyone has heard of helmets for babies with misshapen heads, and a lot of people are afraid their baby will need one. But they're pretty uncommon—I see less than one baby each year who needs one.

Can I give my baby some Tylenol after her vaccines?

Many clinics used to automatically give infants some acetaminophen with vaccines just to make them happier over the following hours. A 2009 study,[24] however, suggested that giving acetaminophen after vaccinations might make them less effective. Perhaps your baby's body needs to "rev up" a bit after vaccines to form a good response. And maybe low-grade fever is a sign of that happening. So, bottom line, I tell parents to hold off on the automatic Tylenol with vaccines. If my kid was really upset later that night and having a hard time sleeping, I'd probably give her some at that point.

How should I take care of my son's penis?

This comes up a lot. For uncircumcised boys, you don't have to do much at all. Don't worry about pulling the skin back. When you give him a bath, water will get in there and keep things clean. If the tip of the foreskin gets irritated (often from sitting in a dirty diaper for a bit too long), a little Vaseline or Aquaphor works wonders.

Circumcised boys require a bit more vigilance at this age. They're starting to get a little "fat pad" on top of their pubic bone, just above the penis. This tends to push the remaining skin forward toward the tip of the penis—sometimes it's completely buried in there! But this skin is *sticky*, and it can sometimes stick to the tip of the penis. These are called adhesions and they're a major pain. You can prevent them by pulling your boy's foreskin down, toward his body (firmly—you won't hurt him), once a day during a diaper change and cleaning away the white gunk that accumulates. (Fun fact: That gunk is called *smegma*, which is just a collection of dead skin cells and oils.) If the skin has stuck onto the tip of the penis, don't panic. Just apply downward pressure a few times per day and it should gradually separate. When it does, put some Vaseline there for a few days so that it doesn't stick again.

My baby's back always pops when I pick her up. Is something wrong? Does that hurt her?

Babies can be remarkably poppy. You can often both hear and *feel* the pops. The most common places are the knees, back, and shoulders. This is totally normal. Your baby has really loose joints, and the ligaments and tendons at those joints often slide over the bones. This doesn't hurt your baby and happens less and less as she grows and those ligaments tighten up. You've probably found that as you get older your body starts to crack and pop again for other reasons!

The only place we worry about popping is at the hips. You've probably noticed your pediatrician kind of aggressively pushing your baby's legs around. We're looking for something called hip dysplasia, where the hip joint isn't formed well. These hips can have some pretty impressive pops and clicks, which need to be addressed. Fortunately, this is rare.

Four Months

Okay, this is getting good. Your baby is a full-on real person now. He doesn't just look at you from time to time—he is utterly obsessed with you. He's desperate for your attention and can't wait to see what you might do next. You could raise your eyebrow and he'll break into a smile. No one's been this excited about you since your parents when *you* were this age (and maybe your partner on your first few dates). And he's not fussy anymore! Unless he's hungry or sitting in his own poop, he's happy and ready to party. There's a ton to talk about. Development is taking off, and big-time changes are happening with sleep and feeding. Let's get into it.

WHAT YOUR BABY SHOULD BE DOING NOW

As I already mentioned, your baby should be crazy about your face. He should smile all the time and maybe even start giggling a little bit. He might be starting to make some "babbling" sounds too, like "b," "g," and "m."

He should finally be getting some control of his arms—realizing that they are attached to his body. Up until now he's kind of batted at things and grabbed them if he happened to catch them.

But now he should be *intentionally* reaching for things like your hair or a rattle. He'll grab them and probably bring them toward his mouth.

Your baby should have pretty good control of his huge head by now. During tummy time he should be able to raise his head up to ninety degrees for a while. When you hold him upright, he should no longer look like a bobblehead.

Should your baby be rolling over? In training, I had always learned that babies roll from tummy to back around three months and from back to tummy at four months. It didn't take me long to realize that this isn't true. Maybe half of kids are rolling by four months, usually from tummy to back first. I'm happy if they can get to their side or get their hips over. Babies in bulky cloth diapers can have a tougher time as well.

Finally, your baby should be excited about putting weight on his legs and bouncing around a bit. And it's quite normal if he's always on his toes or seems really bow-legged while he's doing this.

MUSHY PEAS AND FOAMY MEATS!

Most people are excited to start solid foods, but when can you do it? Well, it's a little complicated. We used to worry that starting before six months put kids at risk of developing more allergies as they get older. Now, most of the evidence suggests that starting a bit earlier can actually decrease the risk of allergies. We also now know there's a "flavor window" between four and seven months where infants are more willing to try different flavors and more likely to retain those preferences as they get older (see Bee Wilson's book *First Bite*[25] for more on the fascinating ways our taste preferences develop from birth). On the other hand, there's evidence that babies who only get breast milk until six months get fewer illnesses than those who get solids before six months. *So I basically think you can't go wrong starting anywhere between four and six months*. There are two things I look for to know when a baby

MAKING YOUR OWN BABY FOOD

I'm always super impressed when parents are able to do this. It's awesome to *know* what you're giving your baby, and I think it's empowering to actually make his food with your own hands. All you need is a powerful blender and some time. You can steam vegetables to get them soft and then blend them, adding breast milk or water as needed. They should be totally smooth. Many parents fill ice cube trays and freeze them for later use. Plastic baby food containers with the snap tops work really well too.

There are some concerns with pureeing your own carrots, spinach, green beans, and beets, because these can sometimes have high levels of nitrates in them. Nitrates can be toxic in large amounts and cause a condition called *methemoglobinemia*, which reduces the oxygen in your baby's blood. Big manufacturers can screen for nitrates, but you can't. I think that having two ounces of home-pureed carrots once a week is quite safe, but if your baby *loves* them, you might want to consider buying those. Also, most of my parents who make their own baby food find it hard to get the right consistency with meats using a home blender. So they tend to buy those instead.

is ready—he needs good head control, and he should be showing some interest when *you* eat. This isn't really a subtle thing—his eyes will get big, and he'll watch you put food into your mouth. He'll lean forward and squirm like he wants to jump off your lap.

Your baby does *not* have to be sitting up by himself yet to start feeding (that comes at six months or later). You can just hold him in your lap. Also, babies have a "tongue-thrust" reflex up until about four months old that causes them to push the spoon out of their mouth with their tongue. If your baby still does this when you try solids, wait a couple of weeks before trying again.

There are some general guidelines to help you with feeding in the first few months, but no exact right way to do it. Baby cereal (rice or oatmeal) is the traditional choice, and I think a reasonable one for the first five days or so. It's an easy texture and unlikely to cause allergic reactions. Also, these cereals are fortified with iron and have been shown to reduce the risk of anemia in babies, particularly those who are breastfed.[26] Full-term babies are born with some extra reserves of iron, but they don't get a lot of new iron from breast milk (formula is fortified with more). So by four to six months, they start to run out of their stores. If they don't replace the iron, babies can get anemic. If your baby (or you) is not wild about cereal, you can add some of the flakes to other purees over the next few months or focus a bit more on meats (see below). If your kid isn't into solids at all after six months, talk to your doctor about whether he might need an infant vitamin with some extra iron.

You can start right away at two solid feedings per day. This should be when he's far enough past his last milk feeding to be interested (maybe two hours), but not frantic with hunger (he'll be frustrated because getting calories into his body with solids is very slow compared to drinking). Just heat up two ounces of breast milk or formula and gradually add more cereal until you get the right consistency (barely sticking to the spoon but way more runny than oatmeal you would eat). Your attitude toward these feedings should be *totally* relaxed. They're just for fun, and your baby isn't depending on these calories yet. Some days he'll gobble down the whole two ounces. Other days he may take one bite and then be more interested in blowing chunky rice spit bubbles. Excellent.

After he seems comfortable with cereal, you're ready for other "stage one" foods, which are single items that are totally pureed. I do think it's really important to establish some vegetables before moving on to fruits. Why? Because veggies don't taste nearly as good as the fruits, but they're more important for the vitamins they contain. Try baby peaches yourself and then try to eat baby green beans without gagging. Fortunately, your baby has no idea that fruits even exist! So he'll usually be happy to try squash, peas, carrots, green beans, and sweet potatoes first. Taste preferences are fascinating—there's good evidence that what moms eat during pregnancy helps determine what their babies like to eat.[27]

Also, remember that meats are considered to be a "first food" right along with veggies. Do *not* taste it, and avoid looking at it for a prolonged time—just the thought of foamy pureed beef almost triggers a gag reflex for me. But it's high in protein and iron, and actually pretty easy to digest. Once you've gone through a few veggies or meats, then you can certainly move on to fruits. His "meals" could then become a bit more complex—carrots followed by plums, for example.

Most babies won't take much more than two ounces of solid foods per feeding before six months. But what if your baby is super excited about solids? How much is too much? He could take up to four ounces of solids twice a day and still have plenty of room to get what he needs from breast milk or formula.

I want to wrap up with a really important point. You'll always have a strong urge to feed your child even when he's not interested. This creates the potential for stress during meals. He'll sense this stress, start to fight feedings, and might even develop an "oral aversion," where he gags when you try to put things in his mouth. So stay relaxed and follow your baby's cues—don't force it.

THE PASSING OF PEANUT PARANOIA

Peanuts are a hot topic right now. I previously told parents to hold off on introducing peanuts and other nut products until after age one due to the risk of allergy. But things are changing. Peanut allergy is a huge problem—nearly 2 percent of kids have it, it's often lifelong, and it can be more severe than other allergies. About a decade ago, scientists realized that peanut allergies were skyrocketing after recommendations to avoid peanuts in at-risk kids for several years. They also noticed that in Israel, where infants universally get fed these little puffed peanut snacks, peanut allergy is rare. Hmm . . .

The LEAP study (Learning Early About Peanut allergy),[28] published in 2015, looked at infants older than four months who were at a high risk of peanut allergy. They found that those regularly given peanut through infancy and toddlerhood had 86 percent less peanut allergy than those who avoided it. That's huge!

Putting these findings to use has been daunting, because it was unclear whether babies had to get allergy testing before eating peanut for the first time. In early 2017 the AAP finally issued some reasonable guidelines that stratify infants into three risk groups:

1. SEVERE ECZEMA (OR EGG ALLERGY). These babies have itchy red rashes that are hard to control, even with the use of strong steroid cream. Kids in this category should get allergy testing at four to six months, preferably skin prick testing with an allergist. If negative, they should be given six to seven grams of peanut protein over three or more feedings per week.

2. MILD TO MODERATE ECZEMA. These kids have rashes that come and go but can be controlled with lotions and weaker steroids. They should consume peanut products starting at six months. The first dose should be small and careful, but no testing is needed beforehand.

3. EVERYONE ELSE. The remainder should be offered peanut products "in accordance with family preferences and cultural practices." A very sensitive statement for those of you with deep family peanut traditions. They just mean treat it like other foods.

So what is six to seven grams of peanut protein equivalent to, and how exactly are you supposed to get it into your kid? Peanuts are a choking hazard and peanut butter is too thick. Try mixing two teaspoons of creamy peanut butter with two teaspoons of warm water until it is nice and soupy. You can then feed this to your baby directly or mix it with some cereal.

THE ORGANIC QUESTION

This is a big decision, and I'll give you my two cents. Organic means food that hasn't been genetically modified and is grown without the help of pesticides, synthetic fertilizers, antibiotics, or hormones. I think there are two main reasons why people choose organic. One is to be healthier, based on a fear that pesticides or modified foods could be harmful. The other reason is an environmental or ethical one—a concern about the effects that pesticides or modified foods could have on the world around us. There is also the concern about how we treat the animals that we eat.

What does science tell us? A few things. Clearly pesticides are dangerous in significant amounts. Field workers with regular pesticide exposure have been found to have higher rates of cancer. A 2010 study[29] in the journal *Pediatrics* found a correlation of higher pesticide levels in the urine of children (presumed to be from mostly dietary sources) with increased ADHD risk. A 2015 study[30] in *Pediatrics* suggested that kids exposed to home insecticides had increased risks of developing leukemia or lymphoma, and those exposed to herbicides had increased risk of leukemia. These are not conclusive studies, but it makes sense that developing brains and bodies might be more vulnerable to harmful chemicals than fully grown ones.

So what if you want to minimize your child's pesticide exposure? Some fruits and vegetables absorb more pesticides than others so that even washing can't remove them all. The Environmental Working Group is a non-profit organization that looks at pesticide levels in foods and compiles a yearly list of those with the highest levels called the "Dirty Dozen." Ideally, these are the items you want to buy organic. Here is the 2017 list (yes, it's more than a dozen, but the name has a nice ring to it):

1. Strawberries
2. Spinach
3. Nectarines
4. Apples
5. Peaches
6. Pears
7. Cherries
8. Grapes
9. Celery
10. Tomatoes
11. Sweet Bell Peppers
12. Potatoes
13. Cucumbers
14. Cherry Tomatoes
15. Lettuce

They also publish a list called the "Clean Fifteen," which as you can imagine features produce that tends to have lower levels of pesticides (even conventionally grown):

1. Sweet Corn
2. Avocados
3. Pineapples
4. Cabbage
5. Onions
6. Frozen sweet peas
7. Papayas
8. Asparagus
9. Mangos
10. Eggplant
11. Honeydew melon
12. Kiwi
13. Cantaloupe
14. Cauliflower
15. Grapefruit

I like these lists—I think they are a reasonable place to start if you're trying to make good decisions for your family but are restricted from buying all organic due to cost or availability. Fortunately, the cost gap is narrowing due to more demand for organics. The USDA estimates that organic produce sales almost tripled from $5.4 billion in 2005 to $15 billion in 2014. Farmers' markets that offer many organic options have also spread over much of the country.

What about things like dairy and meat? I think that's more of a personal preference rather than a choice that will directly affect your child's health. For example, bovine growth hormone given to help some dairy cows produce more milk is not active in our bodies. And while organic milk and meat have more omega-3s (due to more grass in the diet), it's still way less than what you get in a few bites of fish. So if buying all organic puts a stress on your family's finances, then don't feel guilty about not doing it.

ALL ABOARD THE SLEEP TRAIN

Goodness gracious. If you're one of the lucky few, your baby magically learned how to soothe on his own and sleeps through the night now. But if not, get excited! Your baby is finally capable of soothing himself, and you have the power to make that happen. Maybe he's sleeping in his own crib, in his own room, without "crutches" like swaddling. He's finally ready for some sleep training. There are a number of ways to do this, but most pediatricians agree that some version of "crying it out" is the most effective.

Before I go any further, let me just say that sleep training is more of a personal choice than a medical recommendation. Some people have strong feelings about it. As with anything else, you need to feel comfortable about what you're doing with your baby. I'll tell you why I think it's a great thing to try, but the decision is yours. Sometimes parents aren't quite ready at the four-month checkup, and we talk about it again in a low-key way at six or

FERBERIZATION

You've probably heard of the "Ferber Method." Dr. Richard Ferber is director of the Center for Pediatric Sleep Disorders at Children's Hospital Boston. His book *Solve Your Child's Sleep Problems*—first published in 1985 and revised in 2006—promoted the method of "crying it out" in progressively longer intervals. He has continued to do research on pediatric sleep throughout his career. His theories are the basis of what many pediatricians recommend to parents.

nine months. And guess what? If you never sleep train, your baby will be fine. I promise you won't be rocking him to sleep the night before he starts high school.

So what are we trying to get out of sleep training? The major goal is for your baby to learn the valuable skill of soothing himself. He's going to be upset by a lot of things over the next year (or eighteen!), and having some ability to deal with that is useful. You'll still be helping him along the way. After sleep training, your baby will also get *more restful* sleep over the course of a night. When he wakes three or four times per night, he's not as well rested as when he sleeps straight through, even if he spends the same total amount of time in bed. This is going to affect his mood as he gets older and how short his "fuse" is. In the long term, sleep training will often give your baby a healthier eating pattern as well. From nine to twelve months it's important for your baby to get more and more calories from table foods, which is hard to do if he's getting fifteen ounces of extra milk at night. And while sleep training is really designed to benefit your baby and not yourself, don't underestimate the importance of your own sleep. You are a better parent and partner when you sleep well. Your baby *wants* you to sleep—he just doesn't know it yet.

THE SETUP

First, you need to pick the right time to start sleep training because you're actually going to get *less* sleep for a few nights before things get better, so a long weekend or holiday when you don't have a commitment is ideal. Pick a time when everyone is healthy and you don't have a trip coming up. Once you start the process, you really want to finish it so you don't send mixed signals. Remember, it's ideal for your baby to be in his own crib, in his own room. This is a good time to take away any remaining crutches too, like pacifiers, music, and white noise. If he depends on a pacifier to get himself to sleep, that's great—except every time he wakes up you'll have to be the one to go pop it back in. Once he's sleep trained, you could certainly bring the pacifier back when you need it. And for breastfeeding moms who have woken up . . . (doing math) . . . about 500 times to feed your babies to this point, here is a great time for your partner to step up.

I like to keep it real simple. You can read two dozen 300-page books on this, but simple works. Here are the key steps:

1. Put your baby to bed drowsy, but *not* asleep, after a feeding and your normal bedtime routine. You're a pro at bouncing, shushing, and all the other magical tricks you've learned to settle your baby, but now it's his turn to practice.

2. Quietly leave the room and try to go someplace comfortable (probably not right outside the door!). Take a big breath and get ready for some crying. It's really important to have a clock or watch for this part, because a few minutes are going to seem like an hour. Realize that hearing your baby cry has some pretty profound biological effects on you—it makes your heart beat fast and your blood pressure spike. It makes you *anxious* to not rush in there. Stay strong.

3. Wait three minutes, then go in and see your baby for a *very* brief time, like ten seconds. Pat him a couple of times, say a few sweet words, and then get out of there. Don't pick him up or feed him! This lets him know that you're still there, and it lets you know that he's doing okay and didn't get his chubby leg caught between the crib slats.

4. Then add three more minutes to your wait before going in each subsequent time. So on the first night you'll go in after three, then six, then nine, and then twelve minutes. Cap it at twelve minutes for the first night—keep going in every twelve minutes until your baby gets himself to sleep, staying for only ten seconds or so at each visit.

5. Every time he wakes up again later that night, repeat the whole process, going in after three, then six, then nine, and finally every twelve minutes until he settles himself to sleep again.

6. When *should* you actually feed him? Eight to ten hours after he goes down for the night. So if your baby falls asleep at 8 p.m., he's probably ready to eat when he fusses at 5:30 a.m. Most babies will feed and then go right back down for a one- to two-hour top-off.

7. The next night, shift everything back three minutes for all the wake-ups. So you'll go in after six, then nine, then twelve, and finally every fifteen minutes until he settles himself. Each night, you continue to move your intervals back by three minutes, capping it at the fourth interval. Here's a little chart to help you out:

MINUTE INTERVALS

	1st Time	2nd Time	3rd Time	4th+ Time
Day 1	3	6	9	12
Day 2	6	9	12	15
Day 3	9	12	15	18
Day 4	12	15	18	21
Day 5	15	18	21	24

Remember, there's nothing magical about these intervals—as long as you're waiting longer in between visits with each wake-up and maybe stretching it out a bit each day, you'll be great.

THIS IS REALLY HARD!

I had already been giving sleep-training advice for a few years before my son was born and thought of myself as an iron-clad sleep-training machine. But that fantasy died real quickly when we started to do it with him at four months. It was tough! Turns out your baby's crying is perfectly designed to stress you out. Sitting awake at 2 a.m. listening to him scream for an hour was not fun. But after three nights it ended, and he's been a consistent sleeper ever since. Most babies come around within a week. So hang in there, and probably don't listen to a pediatrician in his twenties who doesn't have any kids yet.

You may be wondering: Will your baby hate you in the morning? Is this going to make him a sullen teenager with security issues? No! A 2012 study[31] followed sleep-trained infants until age six and found no differences compared with kids who were not sleep trained. Maybe not surprisingly, the moms of the sleep-trained infants had better sleep and less depression. Be confident in the hundreds and hundreds of hours of bonding you've done with your baby. Really, I think a lot of parents underestimate the strength of that connection. The worst thing that can happen is he might be a bit hoarse for a day. Definitely don't worry that he's hungry—he'll easily make up the calories in the daytime.

SLEEP TRAINING TROUBLESHOOTING

1. It's been a week, you've been religious about your intervals, and things are *not* improving. This usually means one of two things. First, there are a few babies who aren't quite ready to soothe themselves at four months. So think about stopping for now and trying again in a few weeks. Second, some kids are just intense—they're so pissed off when you come in to see them and then leave that the intervals make them madder. If these babies are over six months old, I usually recommend open-ended crying after a week of intervals. Seems mean, I know, but it works.

2. Your baby cries so hard he vomits, or he enjoys pooping at night. These are tough, but just try to clean him quickly and quietly and push through. Your baby probably poops at night because he's used to feeding during the night. He's going to get those calories during the day now and his poop schedule will likely follow. For vomiting, it's okay if you spend some extra time calming him down or decreasing your intervals for a night. If the vomiting happens for a few nights in a row, consider holding off on your sleep training for another month.

3. You only have one bedroom in your home so he has to stay with you. This makes the training more difficult, but it can still be done. Try to put the crib as far away from your bed as you can and then hang a blanket or set up one of those fold-out screens between the crib and your bed. Hopefully you can do the first couple of training sessions each night before you've gone to bed. You can also temporarily use a bathroom or a large closet to ease the process.

4. You don't feel like you're quite ready yet. Could you do it later? Absolutely. You can really do this at any age. But I think it gets tougher after nine months. Remember that your baby will then be standing up and shaking his crib rail. It's a bit harder to settle down from that, so the whole process might take longer and be more emotionally charged for everyone.

WAYS TO GIVE YOUR BABY A BOOST

Over the next few months your baby is going to work on getting a strong trunk (abdomen, back, and sides). Tummy time is always great, but you have some other options now. Infant activity centers, jumpers, or sitting chairs are great places for your baby to hang out for a bit while you get some things done. They partially support his trunk but still let him flop around to work on those muscles. They also let him push with his legs and get even better at reaching for things.

Your baby is going to get really excited about grabbing just about everything and shoving it into his mouth. He wants to learn how to rotate things in his hands and move them from one hand to another. He's also starting to learn a lot more through touch, so letting him feel all sorts of textures—wet, sandy, smooth, rough, crinkly, slippery, bumpy—is really fun.

Your baby even gets a kick out of his *own* face now! Mirrors are exciting. He'll start to respond to sound, so it's a great time to expose him to music. And never stop talking. Since your baby can see colors better now, he'll like being outside even more. Plus, outside is a great place to narrate what you see and touch.

FAQS

How long should I wait between offering my baby new foods? And how will I know if he is allergic to something?

You can introduce new foods every two or three days. If your baby does have a bad reaction, that lets you pin down the new food that caused it. Realize that food allergies to "first foods" are very uncommon. A few different things could happen if your baby is allergic. He could get a rash, usually hives (or welts) that are raised off his skin and can be smaller than a pencil eraser or bigger than your hand. This usually appears within hours of starting a new food. He could also get digestive symptoms, such as vomiting within thirty minutes of eating something. Allergic vomiting is way more intense than spitting up, with repeated retching and a very unhappy kiddo. Lip-swelling and trouble breathing are really severe signs of food allergy, but that would be quite rare with these foods.

Some of my friends are doing "baby-led" feedings. That sounds kind of cool. Can I try that?

If you want, but let's talk about it a bit. Baby-led feeding (also called baby-led weaning) is a fairly recent term for allowing infants to skip the whole puree thing and start feeding themselves by hand as early as six months. While parents are still obviously in control of what is offered, it is usually what the rest of the family is eating. The baby then decides what and how much he will eat.

There really isn't a lot of great research in this area. The term seems to have been coined in the 2008 book *Baby-Led Weaning: Helping Your Baby to Love Good Food*. The authors drew on a very small, unpublished study they had done as master's students a few years prior. They assessed how five six-month-olds responded to being offered small chunks of food while participating in the family meal. Based on this, they concluded that parents should allow infants to lead the way in their own feedings rather than spoon-feed them. That's a pretty big conclusion to reach from such a tiny sample.

Proponents argue that putting the infants in charge will lead to healthier attitudes toward eating and healthier weights since they will be listening to their bodies. I would say that most pediatricians are hesitant about it for a few reasons. First, choking is more of a concern with chunks of food than purees. In a 2012 study,[32] 30 percent of parents practicing baby-led feedings reported one or more choking episodes (most commonly with raw apple). The infants were able to work it out on their own in all of those instances, which likely reflects the strong protective gag reflex at that age. But it still makes me nervous. Also, I had secret doubts about my own kids' intrinsic wisdom as long as they were pooping on themselves multiple times a day, so maybe we shouldn't assume they can take the lead on everything.

I think there are two strong ideas to take away from baby-led feeding: listening to your child's feeding cues rather than pushing, and offering choices. These suggestions can help you grow your baby into a toddler who eats healthily regardless of how you approach solids.

We're vegetarian and planning on raising our baby that way. Is that safe?

It's easy to give your baby good nutrition with a vegetarian diet. There are just a few things you'll have to pay attention to.

PROTEIN. Your baby doesn't need a ton and will get most of it from dairy. Nuts, eggs, soy, beans, and certain whole grains are other good sources.

IRON. I talked about this earlier—your baby needs iron to make new blood cells. Dark greens, beans, and fortified cereal are good options other than meat. You can also consider a multivitamin with iron.

VITAMIN B12. Important for brain and nervous system function, B12 is found mostly in animal products. This is a good reason to give your child a multivitamin if you're raising him vegetarian.

Our baby is chewing on everything and drooling like crazy. He's teething, right?

Probably not. Teeth are unpredictable and can come anytime, but most babies aren't teething at four months. Instead he's using chewing and sucking to explore the world. This excites his little salivary glands and makes a lot of drool, just like teething eventually will.

If we decide to sleep train, should we do it during naps too?

The crying-it-out process can take a while, and it can be tricky to do it during naps because your time window is smaller. But rest assured that if your baby learns how to self-soothe at night, he'll usually use those skills to become a better napper too.

It just kind of happened, but our baby sleeps in the bed with us and I'm okay with that. Do we need to stop?

I always say thanks for telling me. And no, you don't need to stop—remember, you're calling the shots with your baby and your family. But do consider that it's not as safe as the crib for a few more months yet (see page 32), regardless of the precautions you take. Also, don't have any delusions about where this is heading. Your baby is thrilled to sleep with you, and he'll be thrilled to sleep with you when he's one, two, and probably three. If you're not cool with that, then now is a good time to think about getting him into his own crib. Trust me, the battle will be much less intense at a few months old than it will at a few years old.

Six Months

Life is pretty good. Your baby is happy almost all of the time. You've started solids, and that's kind of fun. She has some rolls and looks like she's smuggling grapes in her cheeks. You're a pro at getting out and about with her and are enjoying the little "adventures" you take. You've morphed from beginner parents to experienced parents, and that confidence feels good. Time is starting to pass quickly. You're probably talking to friends with babies and comparing your baby's milestones with theirs; and if you're like most parents, you're probably at least a bit worried that your baby might not be doing everything she's supposed to. What do you say we put your mind at ease?

WHAT YOUR BABY SHOULD BE DOING NOW

Your baby should still be really interactive with you. She should prefer looking at faces over anything else. It should be easy to get her to smile when she's in a good mood.

She should be getting a lot stronger. Some babies can stay upright completely on their own if you put them in a sitting position at this age. She should at least be able to control the top of her body if you help to hold her hips while sitting. Your baby does *not* have to be crawling at this age. She might be getting on all fours and rocking a bit with her butt up in the air, though, kind of feeling it out.

Your baby should be really good at reaching for and grabbing anything she wants. She should also be just starting to transfer things from one hand to the other.

She should be babbling a bit more often and starting to "experiment" with her voice more. This means high-pitched screeches and squeals, low rumbling sounds, and maybe blowing spit bubbles or "raspberries" with her lips.

You might find that your baby is still super happy with you, but not quite as into other people anymore. While you probably could have passed her around a room of strangers a month or two ago, suddenly she might recoil in terror if someone else gets too close. This can even happen with friends or grandparents who she's seen plenty of times (don't take it personally, Grandpa). This is *stranger anxiety* and often starts around six months. Not all babies go through it but many do. It's a normal developmental milestone and just means that your baby has formed a really good bond with you. It usually lasts a few months, unless you are my daughter. Then it lasts from age three months to fourteen months.

Your baby is slowly needing a bit less sleep as she gets older. Most kids will go to three naps around this time. If you haven't done sleep training and your baby is still waking for food or comfort every night, this is a good time to think about it again.

FEEDING UPDATE

If you haven't started solids yet, I urge you to do so at this point, particularly for the iron. If you have started and built up a decent collection of single-ingredient "stage one" foods that your baby likes, you're ready to kick it up a notch. You can start giving her "stage two" foods. These are still totally pureed but have combined ingredients, like turkey and vegetables or brown rice and plums. Sounds tasty, doesn't it? It's still pretty inedible to you or me, but your baby will be thrilled.

Two times per day is still ideal for solids, but the portions can be bigger. Over the next couple months you could let your baby have up to 6 ounces of solids per sitting! (Most kids will still take less than that.) You could also have a few different "courses" at each meal, because it's never too early to introduce fine dining. For example, you could give 3 to 4 ounces of turkey and vegetables followed by 2 ounces of apples and blueberries for dessert. Remember that your baby needs good sources of iron, especially if she is breastfed. She'll get some from any meats, but it's a good idea to still keep baby cereal in the rotation as well.

Yogurt is another option after six months, usually less than three or four ounces at a time. It's a good source of probiotics (live active cultures) and protein, especially Greek-style versions. This doesn't have to be "baby" yogurt, which tends to be more expensive and sugary. Full-fat or at least 2 percent is ideal. The sugar content varies widely in yogurt, so try to find one that has less than 15 grams per adult serving.

There are a few "finger food" options that come into play now as well. You could give your baby rice rusk crackers or teething biscuits as early as six months. They have no nutritional value to speak of, but they're easy for her to hold and dissolve in about three seconds, so they don't pose a choking risk. They can provide a nice ten-minute distraction for your baby if things get dicey while you're out running errands or eating at a restaurant. There are also "puffs," little star-shaped rice treats that dissolve almost as quickly. There are some nice organic varieties of these snacks that incorporate ground-up veggies as well. These usually say "for crawlers" on the packaging, which means about seven and a half months. Babies have a lot of fun with these, and they help with fine motor skills—it takes a lot of practice to figure out how to pick up a small piece of food and get it into your mouth.

A LITTLE TASTE CAN STILL DO HARM

Watching your baby react to little tastes of super yummy grown-up junk food probably seems like one of the cutest things on earth. Parents have proudly told me countless times about how their kids just love to suck on french fries, icing, or ranch dressing. Grandparents seem to enjoy this game as well. A frustrated mom recently told me how Grandpa seemed to bond with her infant son by dipping his pacifier in soda every time she turned around. The problem is, even though these little tastes are just occasional, I don't think it's harmless fun. As I noted in the four-month chapter, we know a lot about how foods your baby is exposed to at this age and even earlier through your blood and breast milk affect eating patterns later on. And I'll save you the suspense—your baby will love anything fatty, salty, or sugary like an addict. Fortunately, she doesn't know those things exist yet, and you should keep it that way for as long as you can. At this point most kids are perfectly happy to get mushy vegetables.

Finally, there are little freeze-dried yogurt melts. These will probably be the best thing your baby has ever tasted because they're so sweet. For us, they were a secret weapon for long flights or "level five" meltdowns.

TEETHING—THE BIGGEST SCAPEGOAT OF ALL TIME!

It's finally time to talk about teething. Many kids will get their first teeth between six and seven months. Usually the bottom two middle teeth are the first to come through. Teething comes like a shadow in the night—no one really knows when it's approaching or what it looks like, but it terrorizes entire villages and leaves only a trail of sleepless devastation. (Was that too dramatic?) Teething will get inside your head, that's for sure. Every time your baby is fussy over the next year, every time she wakes up in the middle of the night for no obvious reason, you're going to ask, "Is it teething?" People blame everything on teething! So we need to demystify it.

Let's start with some science. A well-done 2000 study[33] had parents record eighteen different symptoms as well as every tooth eruption during infancy, so they could see which symptoms correlated. Teething did cause mild symptoms such as biting, drooling, ear rubbing, and wakefulness at night, but did not cause congestion, severe sleep problems, or high fevers.

So if your baby has a cough and congestion, it's more likely a cold. If she goes from having one normal poop per day to three or four watery ones, it's probably a stomach virus. And, as frustrating as this is, sometimes babies are just fussy, or they go through a rough few days of poor sleep for no particular reason. Conversely, if your baby is fussy and pulling at her ears but doesn't have any congestion, it's likely to be teething and not an ear infection.

Let's focus on the fussiness that we know teething can cause. What can you do to help?

COLD CHEWY THINGS. This is the mainstay. They are safe and effective. You can buy a wide variety of hard rubber rings to chew on. Some of these have liquid inside so that you can put them in the freezer or refrigerator to get them cold. Someone will probably also buy you one of those fancy French Sophie giraffes, which is kind of expensive for a dog toy but, hey, it's French. Two of my secret weapons are things you already have at home. Wet a few small washcloths and put them in small ziplock bags in the freezer. Or slice a bagel in half crosswise and freeze it the same way. You can pull these out when needed and your baby can go to town on them—the cold and the consistency are a double whammy of relief for swollen gums.

ACETAMINOPHEN (TYLENOL) OR IBUPROFEN (MOTRIN/ADVIL). You really want to use pain relievers as little as possible for teething. I think they have a role to play, but a small one. Avoid using them during the day, because the cold chew toys work well. If you can see that your baby has swollen gums and she is really having a hard time getting to sleep at night because of the pain, I think it's reasonable to use either one for up to two or three nights while things are at their worst. Remember that ibuprofen can be used only after your baby turns six months old.

NATURAL TEETHING TABLETS. Stay away from these. To many people "natural" or "homeopathic" means safe. To pediatricians those words can mean untested and unregulated. There has never been any evidence that these work. Furthermore, there was a scary recall in 2010 for one of the most popular brands. The tablets were designed to contain a small amount of belladonna, a natural compound that is dangerous at higher doses, but it was discovered that the levels of belladonna varied widely from pill to pill, and there were reports of children suffering seizures after taking them. There was another recall in 2017 due to inconsistent amounts of belladonna. They're just not worth the risk—better safe than sorry.

BABY TEETHING GELS. Also not great. They do work, but the relief only lasts for a short time. The medicated versions contain benzocaine, a numbing medicine known to pose a risk of methemoglobinemia, a nasty condition where your blood can't carry as much oxygen as it normally does. Due to this concern, the manufacturers write "recommended for two years and up" in small print on the back of the box. Yet on the front of the box is an *infant* who looks like he's sleeping soundly. And they recommend using a pea-sized amount up to four times a day. That's a *lot*, resulting, of course, in you buying more. There are also lots of "natural" gels available that are untested and unproven. Again, healthy skepticism.

So when are more teeth going to come? Teeth are kind of wacky! Some babies get their first at four months, and I see plenty who are toothless at twelve months. Teeth will often come out of order with none appearing for three months and then four appearing in one week. In general, most babies get the top four middle teeth next, with six total teeth being about average at twelve months. Then they get the third and fourth middle teeth on the bottom. After that, around fifteen to eighteen months, come the first molars, followed shortly by the canines in front of them. Finally, most kids get their second set of molars a little after age two. If your baby is a late teether, that won't have any effect on what she can eat during the first year.

Caring for baby teeth is easy until twelve months. Just give them a quick five-second wipe once or twice a day with a wet washcloth or baby toothbrush and water. There's no need for baby or "training" toothpaste.

SAFETY AND CHILDPROOFING

Every year it seems like there are more safety recommendations that make it harder to have fun with your child. I also feel like a hypocrite preaching about safety since I never wore a bike helmet until I was twenty and have fond memories of flopping around unrestrained in the family station wagon. But I've also seen plenty of scary accidents and injuries in young kids. So let's talk about a few ways to childproof your home that maybe aren't so obvious. (If you don't know that you should install outlet covers and working smoke detectors by now, please return to parenting school.) Six months is a great time to think about childproofing because the next time we meet at nine months, your little one will be on the move. Babies and toddlers have an uncanny ability to gravitate toward the most dangerous thing in the room. I thought about renting my kids out at that age—just release them in your home and they'll identify all the hazards with shocking efficiency!

- Watch out for cords. You should go around your house and look for cords to lamps, toasters, and other appliances that hang down from tables. By nine months your child is going to be drawn to anything that she can pull herself up on, and she'll bring whatever is at the top of the cord down onto herself. Try to pin the cords between the table and the wall. Beware of tablecloths for the same reason.

- Hardwood floors are beautiful but a pain in the butt with kids. They're slippery! Try to have your kid go barefoot or wear gripper socks. Be especially cautious if you have uncarpeted stairs. Fortunately, if your house is like mine, your hardwood floors will develop a coating of scratches and grime after several years that provides exceptional grip!

- Get in the habit of making rounds to scan the floor where your child plays, looking for small choking hazards like coins, beads, fuzz balls, button batteries (*very* dangerous), and little toy pieces dropped by older siblings. Get on your hands and knees and think like a baby!

- We'll talk in future chapters about how resistant your child is to getting seriously hurt from falls onto the ground, but edges and corners are a different story. They load up all the force of the fall into one area and can cause fractures or gaping cuts that need stitches. Think about padding low table corners and fireplace edges—you can buy foam "corner covers" that work well.

- Balloons are no good for little kids, whether blown up or not. Kids naturally try to blow them up and can inhale them when they take a big breath.
- Blinds and curtains usually have a long looping cord that hangs down and poses a strangulation risk. Try to secure it to the top of the blinds with a hook or clip. And never put her crib within arm's reach of those cords.
- Don't *ever* buy those wonderfully convenient little dishwasher detergent pods or those super-strong fun little magnet balls if you have children under age five. Just don't.
- Household chemicals make me nervous, and for some reason they usually come in vibrant kid-friendly colors (like antifreeze and window cleaner). So make sure they are in childproof cabinets or up high. People often forget about securing their garage, so keep it locked with a childproof door handle.
- When you cook on the stove, turn pot and pan handles toward the back of the range so little miss can't reach them as she gets taller.
- If your child spends significant time at a grandparent's house, make sure you give it a good once-over. You don't want her getting tangled up in a doily or finding some old Pez candies from 1973.

WAYS TO GIVE YOUR BABY A BOOST

First and foremost, talk, talk, talk. Remember to narrate what you're doing during the day. Get comfortable speaking in that singsongy voice, even out in public around other people. You're building a brain here—don't worry about what strangers think.

Your baby is noticing other kids now too and probably likes how they move faster and yell louder than adults. Going to playgrounds will give her some eye candy. Stopping by some library story times or doing parent-baby swim or music classes could be really fun over the next few months. Getting together with other parents, even if their kids are a bit older, is fun for your baby and great for you to talk and exchange ideas. Don't expect your baby to interact with or imitate any kids yet, though. That comes much later. She still does her learning through you.

Your baby can't pull herself up yet, but that's not too far down the road. What you can do to help is stand your baby up so that she's leaning against something with her arms (with close supervision, of course). She'll start to feel it out a bit and work on her strength and balance.

If you are at all outdoorsy, I think investing in a hiking baby carrier is worth it. Your baby will be happy to be outside for a surprisingly long time, probably because she can beat on your head or get a chubby death grip on your hair anytime she likes. It's also the easiest way to carry her for any longer outings, and you can fit all your diaper bag stuff in the pouches.

FAQS

I know my baby is old enough to get the flu vaccine now that she's six months, but I'm nervous. The one year I got the flu vaccine was my sickest ever.

This comes up a lot when your child turns six months in the fall or winter. It's important, so let's spend a little time with it. We use the term "stomach flu" to describe little bouts of diarrhea or vomiting. That is *not* influenza. True influenza is a pretty awful virus that can lead to hospitalization for even healthy children. It can cause high and prolonged fevers, coughing, breathing difficulty, and even vomiting and diarrhea in children. It can last up to two weeks, and infants with influenza often develop difficulty with breathing or staying hydrated. The CDC reports that an average of 20,000 kids under age five are hospitalized with influenza each year.

Unlike other vaccines, the flu vaccine changes almost every year. There are many different strains of influenza, and every year infectious disease experts try to predict which strains will predominate during the next flu season. This means that the flu vaccine is more effective some years than others. But it tends to work well for kids, usually in the 60 to 80 percent range. The first season your child gets the flu vaccine, she has to get two shots at least four weeks apart to boost her immune system. After that, it's just one per year. It's a good idea to get the first vaccine before the end of October since influenza can hit as early as November.

Almost every day in the fall and winter, I hear stories from parents about how flu vaccines have made them or someone they know sick. The vaccine that your baby gets uses a dead strain, so it's impossible to get influenza from it. Also, some people have a sense that the flu vaccine is supposed to keep their kid healthier in general, and then they are disappointed when their kid gets hammered in daycare by illness after illness. Remember that it only protects against influenza. There are plenty of other viruses that can make your child sick—they're just a lot less likely to put her in the hospital.

In making any medical decision, it's good to look at the risks versus the benefits. The flu vaccine should be an easy call. Yes, your child could get a fever or some redness on her leg from it as with any injected vaccine, but even those side effects are rare. I have never seen any serious side effects from *thousands* of flu vaccines. Ever. But I see lots of bad influenza every year, including kids who end up in the hospital. Quite simply, your child is safer each winter with the flu vaccine than without it. As always, decide what feels right for your child, but I strongly encourage getting it.

Someone told me that crawling is important for babies to learn other stuff like reading. Is that true?

This is a myth that's been around for nearly a century, since the psychologist Arnold Gesell published his landmark schedule of developmental milestones and felt that crawling was a crucial one. There are a handful of studies, most of them over twenty-five years old, that suggest kids who crawl develop better social skills, spatial skills, reading skills, and even better binocular vision. Some have even said that "cross crawling," where infants put one arm and the opposite leg forward at the same time, is crucial for proper brain connections to form.

But, non-crawlers assessed in the above studies included a higher percentage of children with other developmental delays, which might explain why they did more poorly on later tests. There's no evidence that failure to crawl is what *causes* later delays versus kids who do crawl. The American Academy of Pediatrics found no basis whatsoever for the brain "patterning" theory touted by proponents of cross crawling.[34] Being a pediatrician, I see so many kids who don't crawl. As long as you give them some time on the ground, they're going to explore the world around them by scooting, army crawling, or rolling. Could you even force your infant to crawl anyway? No. So I don't even ask about crawling as a milestone—I ask about pulling up to a standing position around nine months, because that puts babies on a pathway to walking.

You said we might be able to start a few table foods before we see you at nine months. Are there any foods we have to avoid?

Good question—really just honey. The issue with honey is that it can contain spores of botulism, a super-tough bacteria that can paralyze your child's muscles, including the ones she needs for breathing. Before one year, most babies don't have strong enough stomach acid to kill these spores. I think that the foods on the common allergens list, like eggs, fish, wheat, soy, and strawberries, are fine. If there is a problem with one of these, you'll usually be able to tell before it becomes severe. On page 75, we talked about how starting peanuts early (and cautiously) can reduce the chance of allergy. I tell parents to have similar caution when trying shellfish, such as shrimp or crab, for the first time since it can likewise cause a severe reaction.

We were thinking about getting an infant walker, where our baby sits in a seat and can "walk" around the room. What do you think?

I'd pass on this type of walker, even though we all probably used them as kids. They can be dangerous because kids can fall down stairs with them. The American Academy of Pediatrics has recommended against using them since the 1990s, after thirty-four deaths were reported between 1973 and 1998 and over 20,000 children under fifteen months were treated for walker injuries in 1995 *alone*.[35] There's also some evidence that they can actually *delay* walking.[36] I find it bizarre that they're still on the market.

How about those amber necklaces for teething? I have a friend who swears by them.

These are super popular right now. I see babies every day with them on. Teething can be rough, and parents are desperate to do anything they can to help their babies. But what do pediatricians think about them? That they are cute but a waste of money, as well as a mild choking or aspiration risk.

There are a variety of claims as to how these necklaces might work. Some are downright bizarre, such as that they enable your baby's body to heal itself, radiate healing energy, or harness the power of magnetism. The most rational-sounding explanation is that the amber contains a pain-relieving substance called *succinic acid*, which is released by your baby's body heat and absorbed through the skin. Baltic amber does indeed contain succinic acid, but it melts at 187 degrees Fahrenheit. So your baby wouldn't really be able to melt or absorb it even with a raging fever. And even if she could, would it be good to have a constant stream of an untested chemical leaching into your baby's skin?

There is also a common sense recommendation against infants wearing necklaces due to risk of strangulation. Many of the necklaces are now sold with safety features such as strings that break if pulled on and knots in between each bead so a baby can't swallow a bunch at once. But why take even a small risk on something that isn't effective anyway?

So why do so many people use them? Two reasons: first, your friend telling you that it worked wonders often makes a bigger impact on you than all the stuff I wrote in the above paragraphs. Second, the placebo effect is really strong. If you try something and expect it to work, it's usually going to seem like it's working.

Nine Months

Remember when you could put your baby down in the middle of the floor and casually walk to the kitchen to grab a snack? Well, those days are long gone now. Your baby can probably crawl, scoot, drag, roll, and pull his way across the whole room. He's not quite as easy to keep entertained at this point. He wants everything that he isn't already holding, and he wants to shove it into his mouth. Keeping him happy and busy is a full-time job and can be exhausting. But I'll bet the best part of your day is coming home from work, or waking up first thing in the morning, and seeing your baby smile at you like he's ready to go.

WHAT YOUR BABY SHOULD BE DOING NOW

Most babies are able to pull themselves up to a standing position (or at least to the knees) by now. This is a more important milestone than crawling because babies have to do this before they can "cruise" along objects and finally walk. Babies will usually bounce around in the standing position but haven't really nailed the sitting back down part yet.

Your baby should be better at picking up small objects with his thumb and pointer finger (but not yet with the fingertips). This is going to help him eat small chunks of table food, interact more easily with his environment, and consume various inedible things stuck in the fibers of your carpet.

By nine months, I'm hoping your baby can make some repetitive sounds: "da-da-da-da, ba-ba-ba-ba, ma-ma-ma-ma." (A note to moms: "dada" is easier for most babies to say than "mama," so get that secret practice in.) This tells us that your baby is getting better control of the muscles used for speech, even though we don't expect the words to mean anything. You might also notice that your baby is a bit more into imitating you now when you make specific sounds. And most babies at this age respond to their names, because that means someone wants to have fun with them (but don't expect him to respond right away every time—he'll still get zoned out on something like a light switch).

We've already talked about stranger anxiety, which might still be going strong. Its evil cousin is *separation* anxiety, and it can start around this time. All of a sudden, once-easy drop-offs at daycare or with the grandparents can be screaming affairs. You're playing with your baby on the carpet, step around the corner for a second, and he acts like the world is ending. And sometimes having Dad available isn't quite enough—it can specifically be Mom that your baby is focused on. Again, this is actually a milestone and means that your baby has a great bond with you.

Hopefully sleep is still chugging along. If you did sleep training way back when, I'm sure you've had your baby regress at least once due to teething, illness, or separation anxiety. The problem is, even when the initial issue resolves, he likes that attention and will continue to play you like a cheap fiddle. If this happens, try a refresher course in sleep training—it never takes as long as the first time. Also, most babies will cut down to two naps a day around this age.

Some babies are starting to clap, point, or wave "bye-bye" at this age. But plenty aren't, so as long as your baby still loves to make eye contact and play with you, don't worry about it.

FEEDING UPDATE

It's time for table foods! Good thing, because your baby is probably getting tired of mushy green beans and rice cereal. As with purees, there's no exact right way to do things. We'll just talk about some general guidelines—have fun with it.

First of all, this is a good time to increase from two to three meals per day plus snacks. Solids are becoming a more important part of your baby's diet, and by twelve months we'd like him to get most of his calories from table foods.

Table foods can be scary. If you're secretly terrified about your baby choking, you're not alone. Along with SIDS, I think it's one of the most common fears among new parents, and it can make you reluctant to offer chunks of food. I always try to impress upon parents *how hard* it is for your baby to choke. Babies are born with a really strong gag reflex, so if anything gets near their airway, the surrounding muscles clamp down like a steel trap. This makes babies *gag* easily, where they cough and even stop breathing for a few seconds. Their face can turn red or purple and their eyes can water. Then the muscles relax after twenty to thirty seconds and they're fine. This *looks* like choking but it's not! Be aware that your baby is probably going to do a bit of gagging as he gets used to different textures in the back of his throat. Do stay nearby while he eats and be ready if he isn't able to work it out himself.

You can make choking even more unlikely by keeping the table food chunks the size of a large pea or smaller. Even if it *does* go down the wrong pipe, it won't completely block off the airway like an uncut grape or hot dog section would. The table food doesn't need to be mushy, but it does still need to be a bit soft. Here's a test I like to use to know if it's soft enough: Hold your thumb and pointer finger out parallel and place the food gently between them. If you can mash it without much resistance, it should be no problem for your baby's formidable jaws. Remember that the teeth don't matter at all for eating at this age!

WHAT IF MY BABY IS CHOKING?

I just talked about how rare this is, but it can happen, and parents feel more confident when they know what to do. Clues that your baby might actually be choking rather than gagging include a weak cough, a weak cry, or a high-pitched sound when he breathes in. (If he is crying loudly or coughing forcefully, give him time to push the object away from his airway on his own.) What should you do?

1. Lay him facedown along your forearm or thigh, with your hand under his jaw, cradling it.
2. Give up to five firm blows with the heel of your other hand between his shoulder blades.
3. If that doesn't work, flip your baby back over, still on your leg or arm, so his face is up. Take two or three fingers and place them over the lower part of the breastbone, right below the nipples.
4. Give five quick and firm thrusts down and a bit upward toward his head.
5. Repeat these steps until the object becomes dislodged or your baby develops a strong cough or cry.
6. If he becomes limp or unresponsive, call 911 immediately and look in his mouth to see if you can find the object that is causing his choking. If so, attempt to grab and remove it.

Get comfortable with these steps! Practice on one of your old Cabbage Patch Kids if you need to. If you'd like more in-depth information, look up *Infant CPR Anytime* from the American Heart Association; for a small fee, they'll send you a DVD and a practice doll. Infant/child CPR classes are also available in most areas.

Source: U.S. National Library of Medicine[37]

I always tell parents they can give almost *anything* to their baby as long as it is soft and small (with the exception of honey, of course). But I think some specific examples can build confidence:

- Soft steamed veggies cut into chunks
- Cross-sections of banana cut into quarters
- Grapes cut lengthwise *and* crosswise
- Small pieces of scrambled eggs (a great place to mix in some chopped frozen spinach)
- Small pieces of pancake
- Thin shreds of chicken
- Pea-sized pieces of soft ground beef
- Slightly overcooked pasta, cut into small pieces
- Cooked rice
- Tofu cut into small cubes
- Shredded cheese or string cheese pulled into small pieces
- Black, kidney, or garbanzo beans, lightly mashed with a fork

Herbs and flavorings are fine—it turns out babies like food that tastes good! But remember to keep the bar set low for sugar and salt. If you're making a stir-fry, set aside a little portion for your baby before adding salt to your taste.

As I mentioned, part of giving table foods is letting your baby practice picking things up and getting them to his mouth. That's important, but so is finishing a meal in under an hour. So don't be afraid to sneak in a few bites for him when he's busy unleashing his chubby fists of fury on his food.

Also, it doesn't have to be a clean break from purees at this age! They're still convenient in a pinch and kind of nice to bring on outings. And those pouches are undeniably fun—*I* wouldn't mind trying the organic Mango Kale Quinoa blend. Just be mindful of the sugar content, and don't fall into the trap of giving them at the expense of real table foods.

EAT TOGETHER!

Eating becomes even more social at this age. Try to have your baby sit down with the family for as many meals as possible during the day. He'll notice and be thrilled that he gets to eat some of the same things as you. Everyone's busy, but starting out eating together as a family (around a table without any TV or phones as a distraction) is one of the best traditions you can establish. Studies have shown that kids who eat more meals with their families eat healthier overall[38] and that they hear more "rare" words, leading to higher vocabulary scores when they are older.[39] This is a big-time development "hack," as you tech-savvy folks like to say.

WAYS TO GIVE YOUR BABY A BOOST

As always, talk, read, and then talk some more. Repeat things, get animated, use gestures: "Look at the red car! Do you see the red car? There's the red car!" Since he's getting a lot better with his fine-motor control, it's a great time to let him touch as many safe things as possible while talking about them—things that are hard, soft, sticky, slippery, mushy, squishy, rough, smooth, bumpy, and pokey. He'll start to develop favorites at this age, and he will *never* tire of them. If he gets super excited about itsy-bitsy spider and tries to copy your finger movements, don't hesitate to sing it with him ten (or a hundred) times a day.

Your baby can get around the room now, and he's got places to go, people to see. No time to shoot the breeze. After pulling up to stand comes cruising, where he starts to bravely inch sideways while holding onto something with his hands. He just needs some safe places to do his thing, like along an ottoman or a coffee table away from any corners. You can entice him by putting a favorite toy on the table just out of reach. Next he'll be able to take some steps with help. Your fingers are probably the best thing for him to grab onto, but if you're over three and a half feet tall your back can only take so much abuse. Other options are a push toy that he can walk behind or a little wagon he can hold onto from behind while you slowly pull it. As I mentioned in the last chapter, infant walkers aren't a safe choice (see page 102).

Walking is probably the most compared milestone of all—parents are always asking each other about it, and I haven't met a parent yet who couldn't tell me exactly when their kid started walking. But it's also one of the most variable milestones. I've seen eight-month-olds walk, and others aren't walking until fifteen months (like my kids). Both are normal, so don't worry too much over the next few months if it seems like all your friends' babies are walking before yours.

Your baby is going to start exploring everything and will gravitate toward handles, knobs, and anything else that looks dangerous. It can be frustrating for both of you to always have to say "no" and direct him away from all this exciting but risky stuff. An idea I love is to dedicate one small cabinet or drawer in the kitchen or entertainment center to him. You can put all kinds of things in there that you have sitting around anyway: plastic containers, lids, wooden spoons, rattles, and bright stackable cups. He'll quickly identify this as his special place, and you can redirect him here when he's focused on diving into the knife drawer. Plus you can switch up the objects inside to keep him interested.

FAQS

My doctor did a blood draw to make sure my baby isn't anemic. What's up with that?

Some pediatricians will do a blood test (either at the lab or a finger pinprick in the office) at either nine or twelve months to make sure that your baby has a healthy blood count. Breastfed babies in particular can be at risk for anemia (low blood count) around this age. By far the most common cause is not getting enough iron in the diet to supplement what he gets from breast milk. If the test comes back low, your doctor might recommend giving your baby more iron-rich foods or an iron supplement. Many babies (especially in communities with older houses) will get lead testing at the same time.

Should we teach our baby sign language?

Sure, if you want to. Babies can start to understand and use some simple signs between nine and twelve months. The advantage is that it gives them a way to communicate before they can talk well, which cuts down on frustration. Of course, you're probably pretty good by now at reading your kiddo's cues, so don't feel that you're putting him at a disadvantage if you don't teach signs. If you do it, try to keep it simple with the basics, such as "more," "all done," "help," "milk," "thank you," and "please." I've seen some kids with really extensive sign language systems set up by eighteen months who are not saying much of anything, possibly because they are getting their needs met and don't have as much "pressure" to use words.

Our baby has been turning kind of orange lately, kind of like he has a bad mist tan. Is it jaundice?

My first question is *always* "Does he eat a lot of orange foods?" This is pretty funny. It just happens that babies tend to really love carrots and sweet potatoes, which contain a pigment called carotene. And when your baby eats a lot of carotene it finds its way into his skin and can make it look orange! Especially on the nose and palms. You can tell it's not jaundice because the whites of the eyes don't get yellow at all. And it will go away on its own, unless he's still obsessed with sweet potatoes as a teenager.

We're taking our baby to Disneyland! Any tips for the flight?

First of all, why are you taking your nine-month-old to Disneyland? You realize he doesn't really know what's going on yet, right? And he's way too short to go on the rides. And Mickey Mouse is terrifying when you've got stranger anxiety and . . . Wait a second—are you using your kid as an excuse to go to Disneyland?

Honestly, your baby will probably do just fine on the flight. And if your infant truly enjoys pooping explosively on planes like mine both did, you're going to learn the valuable skill of changing him on an airplane toilet seat during moderate turbulence. I do have a few tips for you:

TRAVEL LIGHT. There are enough logistics to figure out when traveling with a kid. You don't want to worry about how you are going to juggle a stroller and play yard as well. Consider renting a car seat when you arrive and buying most of your diapers and food locally. Borrow stuff if you're visiting family or friends. Think about backpack-style luggage rather than roller bags to free up your hands. Don't worry about covering any contingency that might happen—you're like the MacGyver of parenting by now. You'll think of something!

KEEP THOSE EARS POPPING. Feeding at the breast or with a bottle on the way up and the way down will help your little one pop his ears and adjust to the pressure changes.

KEEP HIM MOVING. I know that the FAA recommends that you buy a seat for your baby and strap him into his carseat during the flight. You do what feels right for you, but that sure can make traveling expensive and difficult. Regardless, he's going to get pretty antsy if he's confined to a seat or your lap for a few hours. So walk up and down the aisles, go back where the flight attendants hang out and bounce around, and even go in the bathroom to let him play with the mirror and water a little bit.

COMFORT ITEMS. You probably would never think of taking a trip without these anyway, but the blanky, binky, tinky, or winky will be a comforting anchor for your baby on the plane and at your destination.

SNACKS. Your child is going to snack a lot more on the plane, which is fine. Snacks are the secret weapon of air travel, so bring lots. You don't want pouches he can slam—you want little pieces of things that take a while to eat. Cheerios, little cheese pieces, puffs, and freeze-dried yogurt melts for code reds. All that eating is going to chew up a lot of time.

MEDICINES. You want to have the basics from your medicine cabinet—acetaminophen, ibuprofen, Benadryl, and hydrocortisone. Many people ask me if they can give a bit of Benadryl during the flight since they know that it could make their kid drowsy. The AAP doesn't recommend it and neither do I, since it would be scary to have a side effect while in the air. Also, some kids have a "paradoxical" reaction to Benadryl where they actually get more hyper. You don't want to discover that on the plane!

My baby grinds his teeth at night. Do we have to worry?

Teeth-grinding (also known as bruxism) is pretty common, seen in about 15 percent of kids. There is a good deal of research about it, but it's all pretty confusing. Some studies have found that children with anxiety are more likely to have bruxism, but there's no evidence that bruxism *causes* such problems. It goes away in most kids as they get older. Also, it's very unlikely to cause tooth or jaw issues like it often does in older people (remember he's going to lose those teeth in a few years anyway!). I do think it's a good idea to let your dentist know about it. And certainly some toddlers grind their teeth while awake just for fun. So, bottom line, if your child grinds his teeth at night but seems happy and thriving, I wouldn't worry about it.

Twelve Months

Congratulations! You made it! Hopefully you had a big party and your baby had a good time smashing cake into her face. Your kid is officially a toddler now, and it can be hard to get your head around that. Toddlerhood is a rollercoaster. You'll probably laugh more every day than you did in the past twelve months. Your child (can't really call her a baby anymore, I guess) is getting more strong-willed and may seem like she wants to do everything on her own. But, to put it delicately, "her ego's writin' checks that her body can't cash." She still needs your help to do almost everything, and her speech is not at all keeping up with her thoughts. So there are going to be some bumps in the road for everyone.

WHAT YOUR TODDLER SHOULD BE DOING NOW

As discussed on page 110, twelve months is an average time to start walking, but even fifteen months is normal. Your baby should definitely be pulling easily to a stand and cruising comfortably around low furniture. She should also be better at lowering herself back down to the ground rather than "plopping."

Most kids will be learning words quite slowly over the next few months. The hope is that maybe one or two words mean something at this age (usually dada or mama), but I don't worry at all if nothing is specific yet. I'm much more concerned that your child makes good eye contact and loves interacting with you. When faced with an unfamiliar person or place, she should also look to you to see what you think about things. Most kids are working on their pointing, which really helps them to communicate what they want while they're working on the words. Comprehension, which you could call receptive language, develops well before speech. You've probably noticed your toddler responding to more words than just her name already.

Your child should now easily pick up little things, even as small as a grain of rice, with the very tips of her thumb and forefinger. This is called a *fine pincer grasp*. Unfortunately, she'll use this skill to patrol the floor and attempt to eat a variety of debris that's hard for you to see from five or six feet up.

Your doctor will likely give you one or two developmental screening forms to fill out at this visit as well. These are designed to cast a wide net to try to find kids that might have different types of developmental delays. Don't worry if your child is not doing a bunch of things asked about on the form—the screenings are useful, but what we talk about in the room is always much more important to me.

FEEDING UPDATE

Your toddler is probably getting more calories from her table foods than her milk or formula now. Eating should be fun, and she should eat when you eat for the most part. She still needs foods to be soft and small because molars are a few months away. But no more restrictions! Even honey is good to go now.

Before twelve months, most kids eat pretty much the same amount every day, and they're not usually too opinionated about what they are served (hence the ability to have breast milk for about three thousand consecutive meals). But toddlers eat differently. First, you'll notice that how much your child eats will vary drastically from meal to meal and day to day. She might just pick at her food for two days, making you wonder how she could have enough energy to play. Then she might be a bottomless pit for a few days. Growth is kind of a herky-jerky process. But when you step back and look at how much she's eating over a longer period, like two weeks, it's remarkably consistent.

Your child will also start to show ridiculous shifts in her food preferences. Maybe she's always liked peas so much that she quivers with excitement when she sees them coming. And then BAM! The *very next day* she gags at the mere sight of them and swipes them off the table, offended that you would even offer them to her. Then one month later she loves them again. Don't worry. She's just testing out that strong will she's developing. So try to keep it interesting, and don't give up on things she's rejected a few times.

What I really want you to get comfortable with is that your child's body knows how many calories it needs to thrive, and it's going to get them. You have to be confident in that. So this means that you don't have to push too hard on those days when she doesn't seem very hungry! Don't get into the habit of making her "clean her plate." Bad things happen when eating gets stressful (such as unhealthy attitudes towards eating, overeating, and oral aversions), so keep it fun and follow her cues.

GOT MILK?

There's plenty to say about milk. Cow milk becomes a perfectly good (and much cheaper than formula) substitute for formula or breast milk at this point. It should be whole milk because your child's rapidly growing brain appreciates the extra fat. Of course, this doesn't mean that you have to stop breastfeeding. You've already given your baby the bulk of the amazing benefits, but continue as long as the two of you are still enjoying it. Do give vitamin D, however, until you switch to cow milk.

When you do start cow milk, realize that it can take a week or so for her tummy to adjust. She might be kind of gassy or constipated during this time. You can make the transition easier by doing it gradually: start out by combining five ounces of formula or breast milk with one ounce of cow milk in a bottle. Then, after one or two days, give four ounces of formula or breast milk with two ounces of cow milk. Continue ounce by ounce until you're at all cow milk.

There's no exact "right" amount of milk, but sixteen ounces per day is a great ballpark. I'm more worried about kids getting *too much* milk rather than too little. A lot of kids love milk and, as they get pickier with foods, the milk intake tends to creep up. This is bad for a few reasons. First, it can cause your toddler to become anemic (which we've talked about before) by limiting the amount of iron she gets from table foods *and* making that iron more difficult to absorb. Second, your kiddo needs a certain amount of calories per day, and when more of those calories are from milk, fewer are needed from table foods. So it will allow her to be pickier. Finally, milk can be pretty constipating, and you don't want to go down that road.

What if your toddler won't take milk or doesn't get anywhere near sixteen ounces a day? No problem. We can work around that. There's nothing magical or essential about milk—it's just a reliable way of getting fat, protein, calcium, and vitamin D every day. A balanced diet should take care of the fat and protein. Cheese and yogurt should take care of most of the calcium, and you can top it off with some beans or dark greens. But you will need to give some vitamin D either alone or in any standard multivitamin, since sunlight and fortified milk are the only other reliable sources for it.

What else should she drink besides milk? That's an easy one. WATER. Honestly, water is the main thing people should drink. You may hear marketing nonsense about the "natural goodness" of juice, but it offers no benefit for your child. It doesn't matter if it's 100 percent juice or organic. To me, juice and soda are the same because they have the same amount of sugar. Juice just provides some extra vitamin C, which most kids get plenty of anyway. Fruit is an excellent source, because the sugar is diluted by lots of healthy fiber. Juice manages to concentrate all the sugar without any of the fiber. Of course, occasional juice boxes for parties and special events are fine. And if you want to blend your own "juice" with healthy things like spinach and carrots along with the fruit, more power to you. (See more on juice and sugar in general on page 148.)

GIVING HUMPTY DUMPTY A RUN FOR HIS MONEY

As soon as your child starts walking she's going to start falling—a lot. Some of the falls will be backward onto her amply padded bottom, but what about the bad ones? The ones where she is stumbling along on the sidewalk and falls hard right on her head? Few things are scarier as a parent. Should you follow her around with your hands outstretched? Let her figure it out and hope for the best? Wrap her in foam padding? When should you be worried or take her in?

First, let me just say that it's really, really hard for your baby to get seriously hurt from a *ground-level* fall. That big bone on your child's massive forehead is really strong. Falls from a height or onto an edge or corner (the coffee table being the time-tested classic) pose a greater risk. The normal sequence of events is a terrible sound when your child's head hits the ground, lots of crying for five to ten minutes, and a "goose egg." A goose egg is an impressive swelling that appears shortly after a fall and can look like a ping-pong ball under her skin. This happens because there is such a thin layer of tissue over the skull that the swelling has nowhere to go but straight out. The goose eggs quickly go down, but you'll see a fascinating spectrum of bruise colors over the following week. And for the next few years, you'll probably be able to find *some* kind of head bruise at any point in time.

When should you call your doctor or take your little daredevil into the ER? Multiple studies have looked at factors more likely to be associated with a significant head injury such as an internal bleed or a skull fracture. There are a few warning signs to look for:

LOSS OF CONSCIOUSNESS OR "PASSING OUT"—EVEN IF ONLY BRIEFLY. Some babies are so shocked from a fall that they have a bit of a breath-holding spell where they don't breathe or cry for a while (but remain awake) before cutting loose, however. That's okay.

REPETITIVE VOMITING. This can sometimes happen several hours after the fall and always requires medical attention. If your little one vomits just once when she's really worked up right after the fall, you're probably fine, but call your doctor's office to be on the safe side.

A CHANGE IN YOUR BABY'S MENTAL STATUS. This is the toughest one to define; you might ask, "Does my baby even have a mental status?" After a scary fall, it's normal for your baby to be a bit more clingy for the rest of the day and maybe to nap a bit longer than usual. But if she's *lethargic*, meaning withdrawn, difficult to arouse, and not as interested in playing or eating as usual, you need to at least call.

A SEVERE HEADACHE. This is tough for your toddler to tell you, but it will be more useful as your child gets older. If she remains very fussy for hours after the fall, it's probably a good idea to have her checked out.

A "SEVERE" MECHANISM OF INJURY. This could be a fall from a bike without a helmet or being thrown from a car.

When one or more of these signs are present, your child has a higher chance of having an injury *inside* her skull (although the vast majority of children will still be declared fine). When none of these factors are present, she has a very low chance of any bleeding or swelling in her head, and you should be fine to keep an eye on her at home. But please don't keep her up at night or wake her every few hours to check on her—that has not been shown to "catch" brain injuries and will probably just make her more upset.

ALL ABOUT TEETH

It's time to brush those baby teeth for real now, whether she has two or ten. Use a bristle brush like yours and just use your toothpaste. The old wisdom was to hold off on fluoride toothpaste until your kid could spit it out (around three years old). But the American Academy of Pediatric Dentistry recommends starting earlier now since the benefits of fluoride are substantial. Too much fluoride (fluorosis, which can stain teeth) is a problem. The key is using a small smear of toothpaste, *no more than a grain of rice in size.* So when (rather than if) she swallows it, it's a negligible amount.

The official recommendation is always to brush twice per day. I think that if you get a good quality brushing at night between ages one and two, you're doing just fine. (An exception would be if your child is still feeding during the night—then a morning brush would be important.)

So when should your child see the dentist for the first time? The American Academy of Pediatrics recommends a first dental visit by twelve months. I've found that dentists have a wide range of recommendations from six months to three or four years old. I usually cover dental issues myself at every checkup and therefore don't suggest visiting the dentist until two years old, when they can actually attempt a cleaning. Earlier visits mostly involve getting used to the office and talking about good dental habits—certainly nothing wrong with that. Also, I'd like to put a plug in for a pediatric dentist if you have that option. They have extra training on little mouths and they know how to work with kids. It's kind of embarrassing how much cooler their offices are than pediatricians'.

Kids are always asking me why we don't have video games in the waiting room and why we only give out stickers and not free toys after visits. I don't really have a good answer for them.

VACCINE UPDATE

After a lovely six-month break, your toddler is due for a few new vaccines. Let's take a brief look at them:

MMR (MEASLES, MUMPS, RUBELLA). This is a great vaccine. These are severe viruses that used to be common. Measles is a nasty and super-contagious virus that causes rash, fever, runny nose, and cough. It can lead to pneumonia, seizures, and brain damage. Mumps causes fever, muscle aches, swollen glands, swollen testicles, and sometimes infection of the brain. Rubella causes rash, arthritis, and fever, but is most devastating if acquired during pregnancy because it can cause birth defects. These illnesses almost disappeared in the United States due to the vaccine, but outbreaks are now becoming more common as vaccination rates fall. There was a large measles outbreak at Disneyland in 2015 that then spread to other places due to low vaccination rates and the high contagiousness of the virus. There was also a massive measles outbreak in Europe between 2016 and 2017, which was predictable, as vaccination rates have fallen below the threshold needed to maintain herd immunity. There were nearly 7,500 cases in Romania and almost 3,500 in Italy in mid-2017. Multiple children have died, but these deaths were all preventable. Controversy over this vaccine in particular really started the modern anti-vaccine movement. The man who started this controversy is one of the biggest enemies of children's health over the past quarter century.

VARICELLA (CHICKEN POX). A lot of parents don't understand why we vaccinate for chicken pox. It was a rite of passage for us. We all had it by the time we were six, did fine, and might

THE BIRTH OF THE MMR-AUTISM MYTH

In 1998 a British researcher named Dr. Andrew Wakefield published a paper in the *Lancet,* one of the top medical journals, claiming to show a link between MMR and autism. The science in the paper was later discovered to be fraudulent, so the *Lancet* retracted it. An investigation also revealed that some of his patients were recruited by a UK lawyer preparing a lawsuit against MMR vaccine manufacturers. On top of that, Wakefield was in the process of developing a testing kit for "autistic enterocolitis" (an unproven condition he made up), from which he estimated he could make $43 million per year. These were obviously major conflicts of interest. He continues to rant against vaccines to whoever will listen. Vaccination rates plummeted in Great Britain after his study and also fell here in the United States. Measles rates have increased in both countries. The anti-vaccine movement has run with his original "findings" and never looked back.

even have fond memories of other kids coming to play with us so they could get it. But some kids didn't do so well with chicken pox. It can cause skin infections, pneumonia, and brain swelling. Before the vaccine was available, about 100 people died and 11,000 were hospitalized each year from chicken pox. That doesn't happen anymore, and it's a good thing. Some parents want to hold off to see if their kids will get it "naturally," but since almost everyone else has the vaccine, they probably won't nowadays. This leaves children more vulnerable to getting chicken pox when they are older, when it is actually a more dangerous illness. Your child will need one more varicella vaccine at four or five years (which can be combined with MMR at that point), and then she's done for life.

HEPATITIS A. This will be offered by your pediatrician at twelve, fifteen, or eighteen months. Hepatitis A is a virus that can affect the liver. It can cause severe stomach pains, diarrhea, and fever for weeks. It can also cause liver failure. It's spread through poopy hands, which toddlers specialize in. The CDC estimates that cases in the United States have fallen from 31,000 per year when the vaccine came out in 1996 to fewer than 1,500 today. Hepatitis A is also a lot more common in the developing world, so it's important for travel when you get older. Your child will need one more hepatitis A vaccine at least six months after the first one, then she's done forever.

WAYS TO GIVE YOUR TODDLER A BOOST

You can swap the bottle for a sippy cup. The bottle becomes a cavity risk factor after twelve months. But for babies who are primarily bottle-fed, it's also the universal soother for bedtime and naps; this is a big change. As such, now is a great time to start building up *other* parts of a bedtime routine. This might include a bath, snuggle time, reading in a particular chair, or listening to quiet music. If consistent, these will be signals for your child to slow down and prepare her body for sleep. There's no huge rush—you have a couple of months to work on that routine and wait for the right time to bring down the sippy hammer. When you finally do, what if she refuses to drink from it? Be strong and wait her out—she'll give in long before she gets dehydrated.

You can also help your child's fine motor skills by giving her a little baby spoon to play around with during mealtime. She's still going to use her bare hands to actually eat, but poking and prodding with her spoon will help her with other fine motor feats over the next few months, like using a crayon.

Your child's finally old enough to start getting something out of public play areas as well. She'll enjoy climbing up steps with help, using a toddler swing, and going down slides with help. She'll start to notice older kids and learn from what they're doing. During crummy weather you can start to explore the daunting world of indoor play places, from McDonald's playgrounds to children's museums. These places are noisy, crazy, germy, and often expensive, but your child will love them.

Reading can be tough at this age. Your child might throw the book, eat the book, or just want to turn the pages as quickly as possible. Stay strong! Remember that you're trying to expose her to tons of words every day, and reading is a more concentrated way of doing that than regular conversation. It also tells her that reading (as opposed to screens) is the most valuable form of entertainment in your house. She hears you, even when she's ripping off her diaper and running around the room while swinging it like a lasso above her head.

FAQS

I was at the store and saw some "toddler formula" for kids between one and two. The can said it had lots of good stuff for the brain and eyes in it. Should I buy that?

If you could see me now, you would notice my eye twitching a bit. This stuff drives me nuts. There's nothing specifically *wrong* with a toddler formula, but your child does not in any way need it. When she was an infant she had to get all of her calories and vitamins from what she drank, but now she's going to get them through the wonderful balanced diet you're feeding her. I don't like how the toddler formula labeling implies that you're missing out on "neuro" or "immune" support if you don't use it. They're just preying on the fact that you want to give your baby the best in an effort to get more of your money. And now they sell "older toddler" formula . . . I'm sure that "high school" formula designed to boost your kid's SAT score isn't far off.

What about other types of milk besides cow's milk? Are those okay?

There are *lots* of types of milk now. Cow's milk is probably best because it has an ideal amount of fat and protein, while most other types have relatively little. As you can see from the table below, soymilk does pretty well on fat and protein. It has fallen a bit out of favor recently because soy contains some compounds called phytoestrogens that could possibly give too much estrogen to kids. If you do decide to give an alternative milk, just make sure it's fortified with calcium and vitamin D and that your child has plenty of other sources of fat and protein. A quick note on goat's milk: it's quite low in folic acid, so your child should take a multivitamin that has it.

COMPARISON OF MILKS, PER 8 OUNCES
(MAY VARY SLIGHTLY BY BRAND)

Type	Fat (grams)	Protein (grams)	Total Calories
Cow	8	8	147
Soy	4	7	100
Rice	2.5	1	120
Almond	2.5	1	60
Coconut	5	1	80
Goat	10	9	168
Hemp	5	3	140

What about raw milk? Is that healthier for our child?

Simple answer: Do *not* give your child raw milk. It has not been pasteurized, or heated to a certain temperature for a brief time to kill bacteria. Some people feel strongly that raw milk is healthier for kids and that pasteurizing it makes it much less nutritious. There is no strong evidence for this. But raw milk can carry dangerous bacteria such as E. coli, salmonella, campylobacter, and listeria. The CDC reports that from 1993 to 2012, there were 127 reported outbreaks due to raw milk that caused 1,909 individual illnesses, and 144 hospitalizations.[40] This is thought to represent a small percentage of the actual illnesses. These bacteria disproportionately affect kids as well (59 percent of the outbreaks between 2007 and 2012 involved kids under age five) and can cause serious issues leading to kidney failure and other complications.

It's true and scary that foodborne illnesses can happen with a lot of foods from spinach to berries to cantaloupe. But the risk is greater with raw milk. It's terrific to support small local farms, but even if your dairy farmer is a great guy, he can't guarantee there's no E. coli on his animals.

How often should we keep shoes on our toddler's feet?

Not very often. The best way for your toddler to get her sense of balance is to feel as much of the ground as possible beneath her toes; that way she can figure out if she has to put more pressure on the outside or inside of her foot to keep her balance or change direction. She can obviously do this better barefoot or in socks than in shoes. When you do need shoes for outings, try to use ones with soft "moccasin-style" bottoms so she can still get some of that feel for the ground she's walking on. And I know this really isn't my place, but I just can't help myself—don't spend a lot of money on shoes! Yes, they are impossibly cute, but they're also ridiculously expensive, and your kid is going to be growing out of them constantly.

When should my toddler go down to one nap per day?

Every toddler is on her own schedule, but most move from two naps to one a day between twelve and eighteen months. You'll know she's getting close when she starts to occasionally miss one of her two naps. When she's missing one of her naps about half the time, that's a good opportunity to consolidate her two naps into one. If she was napping at 10:00 a.m. and 3:00 p.m., maybe you shoot for 1:00 p.m. Don't expect her one nap to be as long as her two used to be together—she's ready for a little less sleep.

Daycare can pose a particular problem. Many daycares move kids up to a twelve-to-eighteen-month classroom at this age and so they have all the kids nap once per day. This can be hard for the younger kids. What can you do about it? Nothing really—most parents tell me that it works out and their kids often keep their two-nap schedule when at home.

Fifteen Months

I love watching fifteen-month-olds in the exam room. All of a sudden their personality takes off. Some kids are all over the place, climbing up on my chair to turn the light off, running around like a drunken sailor, and furiously trying to play with every toy in the room ten times. Some are playful, doing peekaboo from behind their parents' legs and creeping up to me before rushing back to Mom or Dad. And some look like little scholars, patiently flipping through all of the books and pausing only to give me the occasional stink-eye. I'm sure this wonderful chaos pales in comparison to what goes on in your home. But along with all of this blossoming personality come some new issues and questions, so let's dive in.

WHAT YOUR TODDLER SHOULD BE DOING NOW

Your toddler should be walking now—even if it looks rough. He should be able to squat down as well to pick something up and then stand back up again. When he's just starting to walk, it's usually normal for him to be on his toes for much of the time, or for his feet to be pointing in or pointing out. By eighteen months he should be ironing these things out.

Even though motor skills are taking off, we still don't expect a lot of words. We're looking for maybe four or five that seem to mean something consistently. (Pronunciation means nothing—if it's consistent, it's a word.) Plenty of kids have fewer than that, which doesn't worry me at this point. But even kids with no words should be understanding a lot now. As long as he's not distracted, he should comprehend and sometimes actually respond to things you say, such as "Get your shoes!" or "Where's your ball?"

Your toddler should be comfortable holding a spoon and maybe mucking some food around with it. We don't expect him to actually get a lot of food into his mouth with it yet, though.

He should be starting to show some independence, wanting to do a lot of things on his own even when they are tough for him. He should be getting a bit bolder in exploring farther away from you and may finally entertain himself for brief periods. But he should still be looking back at you when he encounters something new or when he's accomplished an amazing feat, such as pulling every single book and magazine from your coffee table—he wants to see your reaction to know that things are okay. He should also still come running back to bury his head in your lap like a stiff-legged chubby cannonball every few minutes to "check in."

A WORD ON DISCIPLINE

If you're like most parents, you probably have at least a fleeting concern that your toddler might grow up to be a juvenile delinquent. He's throwing food on the floor and giving you a look like "Yeah, I just did that—what are you going to do about it?" He hits and bites and seems to think it's a game. You've seen enough tantrums to know that this whole "terrible twos" thing is kind of a loose term. He pretty much does what he wants to do, and when he hears "No!" he gets a special glint in his eye. Is there anything you can do to stop this toddler tyranny?

Discipline is tricky at this age. The problem is that your fifteen-month-old isn't great at connecting consequences with actions, so it's too early for methods like time-outs. But you still have some options:

DISTRACTION. Use his tiny attention span to your advantage. When he's going straight for the outlet for the tenth time, swoop in excitedly and whisk him away to one of his favorite toys or books. Try the same thing when you see those heaving gasps that usually come right before a meltdown.

IGNORING. This is more powerful than you realize, and I think it's underused. If your toddler is having a full-blown tantrum in a safe place, it's okay to ignore it and let it run its course. You *could* run up and give him a big hug and end the tantrum sooner. But he's going to take note of that and may have more tantrums in the future.

If he throws his spaghetti on the floor, your inclination is probably to be a good parent, hide your frustration, and take the opportunity to do some teaching: "No, honey, we don't throw our food on the floor! Food goes in our mouth. Okay?" Not okay! You just gave him a reaction and turned his throwing food into a game. He's a sweet kiddo, for sure, but he doesn't care for your teaching moments yet. As hard as it is, try to ignore it. He might throw stuff ten more times, but if he doesn't get any response, the behavior will eventually be extinguished.

NEGATIVE REACTION. Use this for the behaviors you can't ignore—like biting and hitting. Your kid is getting strong! I've seen parents with bloody noses from whacks, and bites that have broken the skin, so there's no ignoring that. It can happen just as easily when he's happy as when he's sad. How do you handle it? Again, you may default to teaching mode: "Ow, that hurt Mommy! We need to be gentle." Perfectly reasonable, but it doesn't work! Such a reaction will usually only turn it into a game and increase the behavior.

Your toddler has no real idea that he hurt you, or what that even means yet. His hitting or biting reflect poor impulse control rather than a conscious choice. So it's not really fair to hold him fully accountable for the behavior. But how can you change it? Try this: as soon as he bites or hits you, put on wide eyes with a deep sharp "No!" Then quickly set him down and back away from him. This should be done in a whirlwind. Facial expressions, an angry parent voice, and physical separation from you are all things he understands—and he doesn't like them. These are negative reinforcers and should help minimize the biting and hitting. When it's not the "heat of the moment," work on teaching him how to touch gently and praise him for his good efforts.

SPANKING

Discipline is a pretty personal thing. Spanking is probably the most controversial method of all and the one that parents have the strongest feelings about. It's surprisingly common. A recent ABC News survey[41] found that 65 percent of parents approve of spanking as a form of discipline, 50 percent have spanked their own children, and 26 percent think it's okay for a teacher to spank a child—which is still legal in nineteen states by the way!

These parents are trying to do what's best for their child and instill certain values into them. Most of them note that they were spanked as children and feel like that helped shape who they are today. They notice, correctly, that an unwanted behavior usually stops right then and there when a child is spanked.

As I've said before, it's tough for research to change strong personal beliefs, especially since it's not often conclusive. But for spanking, there's an avalanche of research that's impossible for me to ignore. One such study from 2010[42] followed a huge sample of moms starting from the birth of their children. Children who were spanked more often had significantly increased aggressive behavior at age five, even when differences between the spanking and non-spanking households (economic status, domestic abuse, etc.) were accounted for.

Other research has shown decreased cognitive, or thinking, skills in kids who have been spanked.[43] Kids who are spanked even lose some gray matter (important brain tissue) in the part of the brain that helps them evaluate consequences.[44] They also have more mental health problems and tend to expect the world to be mean to them (called "hostile attribution bias").

It's hard to make definitive statements when talking about raising kids, and I shy away from it. But this is one where I *know* that spanking is not good for your child in the long run. I realize it can be difficult to control the impulse when he is driving you crazy, but please think carefully about this. Ultimately, you want to model that physical aggression is *not* the way to respond to conflict. It *is* quite important to set firm ground rules for your child, so please consider some of the other methods in this chapter and later in the book.

PREVENT PICKY EATERS!

Okay, this is a big one, and one of the most important messages I want to share in the entire book. At twelve months, kids are usually great eaters. They're thrilled to try new things and excited to eat off your plate. But by eighteen months something has changed. That twelve-month-old who was downing hummus and kale with gusto now likes only five foods and deftly picks out any molecules of green he finds. The table has become a battleground three times a day, and you're losing most of the battles. How does this happen? Parents talk about being picky as if it is a trait just like having curly hair or dimples. But I want to convince you that *you* have control of whether or not your kid becomes picky. Well-meaning parents fall into some common traps around this age that have implications for how their kids eat for the next few years. Let's recognize these traps and figure out what we can do to avoid them.

On page 116, we talked about how toddlers start to have big-time fluctuations in what foods they prefer and how much they eat from meal to meal and day to day. But how exactly do they become "picky" by eighteen months? Well, they start to realize that fatty, salty, and sweet foods taste better than foods that are not fatty, salty, and sweet. They start to prefer foods that are carb-heavy and starchy over foods with protein and fiber that might be mushy or stringy. And they're *busy*! Forty-five-minute sit-down meals don't fit their lifestyle. They would prefer to graze on snack foods so they can keep on playing. At the same time, they're discovering their independence—that they can control their environment and you.

The result is that they gravitate toward simple processed foods such as hot dogs, chicken nuggets, and mac and cheese. Snack foods tend to be crackers or dry cereal. Toddlers often like milk because they can pound it and move on—many would live on milk if you let them. Most continue to enjoy fruit because it's sweet. Vegetables often fall out of favor, even when you try to hide them. Little kids tend to avoid meats and dishes such as stews and casseroles that have multiple ingredients (you have to admit, tuna surprise can look a bit suspicious).

Now here's the clincher, the thing that really sets a vicious cycle in motion: It's dinnertime. You've made a wonderful lasagna with lots of good stuff in it—zucchini, spinach, whole wheat pasta, ground turkey. You've even sautéed some carrots on the side with just a little bit of butter so that they are soft and sweet, just how your toddler used to like them. He looks at everything on his plate, scrunches up his face in disgust, and refuses to touch it. You start to work your playbook, zooming the food in like an airplane, taking a bite yourself with a ridiculous smile to show him how delicious it is, even busting out the spoon that looks like a bulldozer. He's having none of it, shaking his head from side to side with sealed lips and whacking the food with his chubby palm like he's trying to kill a fly. You're trying to keep your cool, but it's only thirty minutes until bedtime, so you try to sneak a bite into his mouth when he's not looking. He spits it out, even picking a small shred of spinach from his teeth and flinging it to the floor. You look at your partner with a sigh and a shrug of your shoulders that says, "Well, he has to eat *something* before bed." So in defeat, you microwave some dino-nuggets, which he accepts with a look of triumph.

This is a frustrating scene that plays out regularly in a lot of homes. But it doesn't have to be this way. The key mistake is thinking, "Well, he has to eat *something* before bed." This leads to giving the "fallback" food, which may not be actual junk food but it's still not what you want him to eat. As long as food is available to him, your toddler is eventually going to eat. Maybe not this meal, maybe not even much today, but that drive to get calories is so strong that he will definitely eat before he loses weight.

This means that it's okay for him to miss a meal! I know this goes against many parents' instincts. I often tell parents to imagine offering their toddler a bowl of mushy rice porridge with tons of vegetables, a little meat, and all of the vitamins he needs for every single meal over the next year. What would happen? He probably wouldn't eat it today or maybe even tomorrow. But he'd come back to my office a year later and his height and weight would be at roughly the same percentiles they are now. Of course, you won't give him rice porridge for every meal; you're going to try to meet him halfway and offer him things that look and taste good. But I want you to feel confident and in control when deciding what your kid eats.

When you're using this strategy, your vibe shouldn't be confrontational—you simply offer him a couple of healthy choices, and if he doesn't eat it after a reasonable period of time, he can be done. Don't offer more food options. Don't engage him in a battle. The tone is not, "Fine! If you don't want to eat what I made, then don't eat anything!" (Put that one in your pocket, though. It will come in handy during the teenage years.) Instead, it should be more matter of fact: "This is the way things are going to be, at every meal, always." You can even keep the food there if he wants to come back later. Toddlers may not realize it, but they like consistency and knowing where the boundaries are.

There are a few pitfalls that can sabotage this strategy. Kids are kind of sneaky. Your toddler might try to drink more milk to make up some of the calories he's missing during mealtime. Don't let him—keep that milk around sixteen ounces. He'll also try to increase his snacks—kids can get a surprising amount of calories per day from grazing on crackers, puffs, fruit, and other carb-heavy delights. Keep them in check.

Don't get me wrong—I can tell you from experience that even with this strategy mealtimes are not perfect. Your toddler is still going to eat too fast and then too slow. He'll throw food, shake milk onto the floor, and have a tantrum because he can't use your steak knife. That stuff comes with the territory. There are countless little battles that you have to fight with your independent toddler, and he'll win a lot of them. But *you* should win this one. You should ultimately decide what your kid eats—you set the bar where you want to and he'll respond to it. I'm going to put this in writing now, because when I'm a grandparent someday I'll apparently forget it: don't worry about *how much* your kid eats, worry about *what* he eats.

WAYS TO GIVE YOUR TODDLER A BOOST

Set out a bowl of cereal and a sippy cup of milk, take cover, and enjoy the show. Just kidding. But your kid does need safe spaces to be adventurous and explore. Your job is to set boundaries and save him from himself when necessary, but also to hold back from sweeping in to prevent any small risk or frustration. He's interested in everything and wants to figure out how things work on his own. Try to gently guide him without doing everything for him. For example, when he's trying and failing to get onto a little toddler car, don't just plop him on when he starts to get frustrated. Try swinging his leg over the seat and show him how to put his hands on the handles to pull himself up.

In addition to talking constantly to him, a few strategies can encourage your toddler to practice more words. When he points at something and grunts, you know exactly what he wants. But make him work for it a little bit—when he's pointing at his milk, play dumb for a few seconds and say, "What do you want? Do you want water? Oh, your milk? Do you want your milk?" This both reinforces the names of things and gives him a gentle nudge to realize that he can get things more easily with his words.

Kids at this age also start to become more interested in animals, vehicles, and the sounds that they make. This is a great "back door" into talking. Look through books just to point at animals and make the sounds. Your toddler will love to hear them and will hopefully try to mimic them. Is "*vrooom!*" a word? I don't know, but by practicing sounds like this your child is going to get better at saying other words too.

Fine motor skills are taking off. We've already talked about playing around with a spoon. Now it's time to hand him a big crayon and let him try it out. When he prefers to bang it on paper rather than trying to eat it, you know he's ready to go. Even though he might only be interested for ten seconds right now, soon he should be doing some advanced linear scribbling.

FAQS

Our son has started hitting himself pretty hard on the head. Sometimes it's when he's angry or tired, but other times he does it while smiling. Does he have a complex already?

Toddlers (both boys *and* girls) do all kinds of self-stimulating and self-soothing behavior that can look quite concerning. They can hit their heads, rock, shake their heads back and forth, dig at their ears, and flap their hands. I even had one patient whose bedtime routine consisted of getting on his hands and knees and ramming his head into the rails of his crib until he fell asleep. Believe it or not, all of these things are usually normal! A lot of parents are aware that kids with autism might tend to do some of these things more than other kids. And that's true, but many non-autistic kids use these behaviors to calm themselves, express excitement, or deal with anger and frustration. Parents often unintentionally make it worse by attempting to stop the behavior (which is only natural when you see your child banging his head against the wall). This attention just reinforces the behavior and often results in greater frequency. Just know that he will *not* hurt himself, no matter how bad it looks, and the behavior will usually pass with time.

Our kid *hates* brushing his teeth. It's like World War III every night. Any tips? Can we just give up on it?

There are two types of toddlers in the world: those who love brushing their teeth and those who hate it. There really is no middle ground. Pinning down the screamers is a rough way to start the calming bedtime routine. But this is a battle you should fight, at least to get in one good brushing at night. If your toddler gets a cavity it's a big deal, because his dentist would have to give him anesthesia to fix it. And there's growing evidence that anesthesia is not so great for little brains.

Here are a few tricks that can help: Try one of those little cheap electric toothbrushes for your child (the kind that usually has Elmo or Elsa on it). Kids can hate the violent back-and-forth motion of brushing that jabs into the back of their mouth, but with the electric brush you just hold it in one place while it spins and does the work. This is also a great time for distraction, maybe having one special thing on your phone that he gets to watch only during tooth-brushing time. All you need are twenty to thirty good seconds. Around this age, I started telling my kids little stories about animals made up on the spot, which kept their attention during brushing for the next two years.

When does that soft spot on the head close? That thing still weirds me out . . .

Fifteen months is about average, but a normal range for the anterior fontanelle to close is as early as three months until well after age two. It's not typically a concern if your kid's soft spot is still wide open as long as his head is growing at a normal rate.

"Crying it out" just doesn't work for us, but our little one is still waking up throughout the night. Help! Is there anything else we can do?

Sure, there's always something else you can do. First I'll go on record saying that I think crying it out (which I talk about on page 79) is still the most effective method of sleep training, even at this age. But there is another reasonable option. Rather than soothing your child at increasing time intervals, you can do it at increasing distances while staying in the room with him. First, you sit right at the bedside and soothe with your hands, words, and kisses (no feeding, though). You do this every time your toddler wakes up and you stay in the room until he gets back to sleep. Then after one or two nights you move back to arm's distance. You continue to move closer and closer to the door every one or two nights until you are sitting in the doorway soothing only with a quiet voice. After a couple nights at the door, you're staying out completely. This can be a bit time intensive, but it will hopefully get you where you want to be.

My fifteen-month-old walks on his toes a lot, especially when he's excited. My neighbor said he might have something wrong with his spine. Should I worry?

It's true that walking on tiptoes can be a sign of a spine or nerve problem, but those cases are the exception. Lots of kids walk on their toes occasionally between ages one and two when they're excited or nervous, or just for fun. This usually happens less over time. It's reassuring if they are able to be down on flat feet for significant stretches. Check with your doctor if he does it more than half of the time at eighteen months or if you think it's happening more often over time. Even most of the kids who *are* doing it more often just have tight heel cords that simply need to be stretched out. A small percentage of persistent toe-walkers do have underlying spine issues, but these kids usually have other obvious problems such as abnormal reflexes and poor bowel and bladder control as they get older.

Eighteen Months

Something went wrong at some point. Your kid used to like me. She'd smile back when I smiled and maybe even offer a half-eaten cracker. Her look said, "I'll tolerate you. I realize you have to give me a few shots—I'm not excited about them, but you seem like a pretty nice guy." Now she's having *none* of it. I can't distract her anymore with my party tricks. She pushes my stethoscope away and tries to climb up onto your head to escape my evil hands. Eighteen-month-olds are tough. They notice every detail around them and form strong opinions. And those opinions change from day to day! It's incredible to see how independent and confident they're becoming, and a bit horrifying when you don't really know how to handle that yet.

WHAT YOUR TODDLER SHOULD BE DOING NOW

Your toddler should be saying more words. We're looking for ten to twenty by this time. What counts as a word? Any sound that consistently means something, even if the pronunciation is way off. Probably not animal sounds. "Uh-oh" seems like a word to me. Beyond that, you decide. And *lots* of kids have fewer than ten words. Boys especially seem to take a little longer to get to that point. If your toddler is one of those who is a bit slow on the words, don't worry. *Progression* of language skills and understanding are more important than number of words at this age. So if your kid said nothing three months ago but now says five words and understands everything you're saying, I'm not worried. And I worry only a *little* bit about kids who aren't saying anything! I'll usually recommend a hearing test if that's the case, but the vast majority of those kids will have a language explosion sometime before age two.

Your toddler probably has a little more patience for books now. She should recognize some basic pictures like trucks, boats, and balls, and be able to point to them when asked. She can probably make some animal or vehicle sounds too, which makes reading more fun for her. Some kids are starting to understand more abstract things like colors, shapes, and body parts, but we definitely don't expect this yet.

Your toddler should also be developing some serious physical skills. She should have a stiff-legged run and be climbing well. She should be close to walking up and down stairs one step at a time while holding your hand. She should be able to throw too, usually food, but maybe a ball every now and then. She should have enough balance to kick a large ball forward after you've shown her how to do it. She should be able to actually get some food into her mouth with a spoon (messily, of course). When she holds a crayon, she should be able to do some truly inspired side-to-side scribbling.

Most kids at this age love to help and to imitate you. She might want to help you sweep the floor or pretend that she's fixing something with tools. She might want to hang out in the kitchen, stirring and pouring with her wooden spoons and mixing bowl. She watches you cut the grass and wants to do it to with her little toy mower. She's not just obsessed with your face and your attention anymore—she's paying attention to the *details*. It's cute, but it's so much more than that. Along with her commitment to doing everything on her own, this is how she learns at this age. By observing, repeating, and struggling, she learns motor skills, patterns of movement, and how things work. It's one of the true joys of parenting to watch those little gears in her head turning as she figures the world out.

Now that you're feeling good about all the marvelous things your toddler can do, I'd better bring you back down to earth. Your child should be checking out some other kids, but don't expect to see any real interactions between them besides ripping a toy away from one another. She will be terrible at sharing. For a long time. Toddlers' brains aren't really wired to be empathetic or to realize how their actions affect others yet (see page 172 for a more in-depth discussion of sharing). It doesn't mean they're selfish—it's just where they're at right now. Also, while she's great at *understanding* you, that does not mean she's good at *listening* yet. She will be having lots of tantrums, multiple times per day—it comes with the territory. Many of her skills are skyrocketing, but impulse control is not one of them.

ANXIETY OVER AUTISM

There are a few things that almost all parents worry about in my experience: SIDS, choking, and autism. The concern over autism is understandable because it's more common than we used to think, and there's been a lot of media coverage about it recently. The latest research suggests that one in sixty-eight kids has autism,[45] versus only one in 166 ten years ago. It's clear that part of the increase is because we're better at recognizing and diagnosing autism. But most experts would agree that more kids are developing it now as well.

Autism spectrum disorder actually refers to a large group of brain development disorders. Because it's a spectrum (rather than a condition you simply have or don't have, like a peanut allergy) it can look different in different kids. But they all share some common threads. Children with autism usually have some difficulties in three areas:

1. COMMUNICATION. Many kids with autism do not talk or talk very little, but there is a lot more to communication than speech. They might not point at things that interest them or respond when you point to something. They might repeat certain words or phrases over and over again. They might give answers to questions that do not make sense. At ages two and three, they might have a hard time with imaginative play such as pretending to walk a dog or feed a doll. When they enter school, they can have a hard time picking up on things like sarcasm and jokes. Body language and facial expressions are often lost on them.

2. SOCIAL INTERACTIONS. Kids with autism usually have trouble making eye contact. They often prefer to play alone, but without necessarily "checking in" with you from time to time like most toddlers do. They might not respond to their name like most kids do by twelve months. When they get upset, it might be very hard to comfort them with typical methods like hugs and reassuring words. A meltdown might last for over an hour rather than five to ten minutes as it does for most toddlers. Kids with autism have a hard time learning cues that might indicate how another kid is feeling. This makes social tasks like taking turns very difficult.

3. REPETITIVE BEHAVIORS AND UNUSUAL INTERESTS. Most toddlers move around a room like a pinball, bouncing from activity to activity with a remarkably short attention span. But kids with autism often do one repetitive behavior for a very long time. They might carefully line up all their cars for an hour, or focus on spinning a wheel for thirty minutes. They tend to like things a very particular way—if someone breaks up their line of cars they have a meltdown. They can be extremely picky, only eating white foods with a particular texture, for example. While most kids tend to do better with routine, kids on the

spectrum can *fall apart* if their routine is broken. They often do repetitive movements with their bodies to either calm or stimulate themselves. This can include flapping their hands, rocking, or shaking their heads back and forth.

THE CAUSES OF AUTISM

We don't know the roots of autism for certain, but researchers are getting closer. What's clear now is that there are multiple factors involved. Genetics seem to be the biggest factor. We know this because when one identical twin has autism, the other twin has about a 70 percent chance of having it as well. Studies have also shown that among siblings of kids with autism, 7 to 18 percent will also have it (a much higher rate than the 1.4 percent in the general population). There are also clear environmental risk factors, the most important of which affect pregnancy and the time right after birth. These include older age of either biological parent, stressors during pregnancy such as viral infections or diabetes, and maybe even low oxygen levels after birth. Other research has suggested that chemicals such as PCBs and air pollution might increase risk. So what does *not* cause autism? There is overwhelming evidence that vaccines don't, whether you look at individual vaccines such as MMR, or getting multiple vaccines at once. (See pages 50 and 123 for more on this.)

Now here's the anxiety-provoking part. *Most* toddlers show some of the above signs from time to time. Kids often flap their hands briefly when excited or have a meltdown if someone knocks down a tower they built. They might sit in the corner for thirty minutes obsessing over a remote control. They might not be great at making eye contact because they want to get back to their toys as quickly as possible. So just realize that a lot of these behaviors can be normal—just like with regular development, you have to step back and look at the whole picture.

Your pediatrician should help you by using some simple tools or questions to screen for autism and related disorders several times over the first two to three years. If you are worried, please bring it up! It's hard to get a read on a kid in only fifteen minutes in the exam room, so we rely on what you tell us about her behavior. If your pediatrician is concerned about autism, he can refer you to a developmental specialist who can do some further screening. Autism can't be cured, but therapy can improve social and communication skills substantially when started early. The kids I see with autism are fascinating. They see the world in different ways and, despite their challenges, often have remarkable skills in math, memory, music, and creativity.

A WORD ON SOCIALIZATION

Parents really start to worry about whether their kids are getting enough interaction with other kids around this age—particularly when there aren't siblings at home. Many parents even think about putting their kids in daycare a few days a week for this reason alone, even when they don't need to. This is a reasonable concern, but I think it's useful to understand where an eighteen-month-old is at with her social development. Your child is still learning everything from you. She will observe other kids but doesn't really interact with them in a meaningful way yet. From now until at least age two, she'll probably be engaging in more parallel play, where she's doing her own thing right alongside another kid doing her own thing. They might check each other out a little bit, but they're not sharing a game of Candy Land just yet.

This means that your toddler really isn't getting behind if she doesn't spend a lot of time with other kids. Of course, it's healthy for both of you to get out to playgrounds, coffeehouses, the library, the zoo—places where you both get a change of scenery. From age two to three everything changes: she'll interact more directly with other kids and start the long process of learning how to "play nice." And gradually increasing preschool time from ages three to five will get her ready for kindergarten.

FEEDING UPDATE

There's not too much to report here. If you're struggling with a picky toddler, I'd recommend going back and rereading page 133. If you and your pediatrician feel good about your toddler's weight and the other fats in her diet at your eighteen-month visit, feel free to switch from whole to 2 percent milk. If the rest of the household drinks whole milk, stick with that.

Another thing most parents notice is that their kids tend to seriously gravitate toward carbs and dairy by this age. They do need plenty of carbs, especially those in whole grains (as opposed to processed ones or simple sugars). But getting protein can be a challenge, especially since a lot of kids aren't crazy about the texture of meat yet. Fortunately, there are plenty of high-protein options that kids do tend to go for. Greek yogurt has twice the protein of regular yogurt and usually less sugar. Beans, hummus, eggs, tofu, and peanut butter are excellent sources. Quinoa and other whole grains have a surprising amount of protein. So prioritize gritty-looking bread and whole grain mac and cheese when you can.

LENTILS AS SUPERFOOD

The term "superfood" is abused, but lentils are ridiculously nutritious. I'm an obsessive label-reader, and it's hard to find a food as healthy as lentils. One cup of cooked lentils provides 36 percent of your daily protein needs, 63 percent of fiber, and 37 percent of iron. They have tons of folate, B vitamins, and other essential minerals. Dried lentils are also super cheap, and they come in a few fun colors. They are a great base to mix in lots of other vegetables and meats. Just throw them in the slow cooker and watch them transform. As versatile and healthy as they are, somehow lentils are not very popular! Okay, there is one downside. All that fiber makes for some gassy kids. *Seriously* gassy.

SUGAR, SUGAR, EVERYWHERE

Sugar is on the short list of things I get pretty worked up about. Some is essential for life—evolution shaped us to seek out and crave those sweet high-energy fruits that used to be hard to come by. But sugar is not hard to come by now, and if you don't keep your guard up, your child will absolutely get too much of it. When it comes to sugar, *be skeptical*. It may be very true that the history of soda is all tied up in Norman Rockwell nostalgia, being young and having fun, and polar bears. And maybe grandfatherly farmers in Florida do indeed tenderly pick their own oranges in the morning sun with the goal of bringing homestyle goodness to your child. Or maybe there are a bunch of wealthy folks in suits worried about the bad rap sugar is getting. Maybe they fund lots of research to show that sugar's not so bad. And maybe they've paid large sums of money to get their products into the schools your child will attend.

What's so bad about sugar, anyway?

SUGAR MAKES CHILDREN MORE LIKELY TO BE OVERWEIGHT. A 2013 study found that kids who drink more sugar-sweetened beverages between ages two and five are 40 percent more likely to be obese by ages four and five.[46]

SUGAR MAKES IT HARDER FOR YOUR BODY TO KNOW WHEN IT'S FULL. Leptin is an important hormone that tells your brain when you're sated. But consuming too much sugar can cause your body to become resistant to leptin and miss out on that signal. Then you eat too much, which further increases leptin resistance in a vicious cycle.

SUGAR OVERWORKS YOUR PANCREAS. Your pancreas makes insulin, which is crucial for taking all that sugar from your blood and bringing it into your cells where it's used for energy. But your pancreas is more likely to conk out if it's producing insulin at maximum capacity for years. And that's the first step toward type 2 diabetes.

SUGAR CAN AFFECT YOUR LIVER IN A SIMILAR WAY TO ALCOHOL.[47] There is also evidence that it seems to age your brain cells a bit faster and contribute to problems with memory.

FULL SUGAR DISCLOSURE

I really am a terrible hypocrite. When I was a kid, my favorite candy was Fun Dip (candy cigarettes being a close second). Do you remember Fun Dip? It consisted of three packets of pure fruit-flavored sugar. But that's not the best part. Instead of forcing you to use your finger, they actually gave you two "Lik-A-Stix" made out of sugar to eat your sugar! Oh, the memories.

SUGAR MAY AFFECT YOUR CHILD'S BEHAVIOR. I try to back up most claims with scientific evidence, so I have to be honest that there really is no consistent high-quality research showing that increased sugar makes a child more irritable, aggressive, inattentive, or emotional. But I do have two eyes and two kids, and I'm telling you *it affects their behavior*. Perhaps it's the adrenaline caused by the excitement over the sugar. This is a great chance for you to do some research on your own child! Yay, science!

The American Heart Association recommends that children over age two get no more than 6 teaspoons of "added sugars" (sugars used as ingredients in processed foods) per day. But in a 2012 data brief, the National Center for Health Statistics estimated that children overall get over 20 teaspoons per day,[48] and that children aged two to five get over 13 per day! That's a lot and means kids get about 16 percent of their total calories from added sugar. About half of this comes from beverages, with soda being the biggest single source. Kids who eat more meals away from home have higher sugar intake. It's probably not surprising to you that soda and fast food have a lot of sugar, but it hides in foods you wouldn't expect as well.

HIGH-FRUCTOSE CORN SYRUP

Most people are aware of the controversy over high-fructose corn syrup and the concern that the fructose might pose additional health risks over sucrose (table sugar). This picture isn't quite clear—fructose might be a bit more harmful to your body, but sugar is sugar. The real danger of high-fructose corn syrup over the last forty years is that it has become a cheap way of sneaking a lot of sugar into *many* different foods, and the industry's success is now ensured by powerful corporations, lobbyists, and politicians.

SUGAR CONTENTS OF COMMON FOODS

Food Item	Grams of sugar	Teaspoons of sugar
Apple juice (8 ounces)	28	7
Raisins (¼ cup)	29	7
Yoplait Strawberry Yogurt (6 ounces)	26	6.5
Campbell's Creamy Tomato "Soup on the Go" (11-ounce container)	22	5.5
Ketchup (1 tablespoon)	4	1
Nutri-Grain Raspberry Bar (1.3 ounces)	13	3
Prego Traditional Italian Sauce (½ cup)	10	2.5

Remember, four grams (one teaspoon) of sugar is a packet of sugar. Realizing that you're giving your child nearly seven packs of sugar in one serving of yogurt puts things in perspective. Also, our society has been more concerned with fat in foods rather than sugar for a long time. So beware of products that say "low fat" or "reduced fat"—companies often try to maintain flavor in these items by adding more sugar, which is not a great trade-off for anyone, but especially your kid. Getting familiar with food labels is a great way to watch your child's sugar intake.

POTTY-TRAINING PATIENCE

Is it time to potty train? Whoa there! Just take it easy. . . . Potty training is kind of its own little thing. You have the power to change a lot of your toddler's behavior, eating, and sleep habits, but potty training is different. Your approach should be *super* laid-back. It won't happen until your child is ready, no matter what you do. Ideally it's all wrapped up by age three, but it's not uncommon for it to take longer. It certainly did in our household.

That being said, you can start to set the stage as early as eighteen months. The "way in" is that your toddler really likes to imitate you at this age. Let her watch you on the potty (I promise it won't give her a complex). Let her look into the potty and help you flush it. Use potty language all the time and make it seem normal: "Did you make a poopy? Oh, you pooped!" At least one study found that using negative poop words like "stinky" or "gross" can make potty training take longer. So try to avoid gagging in front of your child when you deal with her poop. Get a couple of toddler potties. Put one in the bathroom next to the toilet and one out in her play area. If she's okay with it, she can sit on the potty (diaper on) to play or read a book with you for a few minutes. When she does poop in her diaper, you can walk over with her and put it in the potty occasionally. Remember, act like you couldn't care less whether she is interested or not. Don't go overboard with the praise when she sits on the potty, either—toddlers have an intuitive potty-pushing radar, and she'll get suspicious.

I talk more about this on page 165, but over the next six months, there are some signs that your toddler might be getting ready for potty training:

- She goes longer in between peeing, like two to three hours. This means her bladder can store more and that the "sphincter" muscle that holds the urine in is getting stronger.

- Her motor skills progress to the point where she can help undress herself and take off her diaper or pull-up. Anytime she can help or do something on her own, you'll have a better chance of success.

- She starts to give more signs that she is about to pee or poop. This can be a grimace on her face, a squirmy-leg dance, holding her diaper, or creeping off to a favorite place. These signals will be important at some point for you to know when to rush her to the potty.

- She comes to you sometimes after she's peed or pooped to let you know. That's a big sign that she's ready to make some progress.

A 2002 study[49] found that most toddlers don't develop the interest and bladder control to stay dry until after they turn two, that kids tend to finish potty training between two and a half and three, and that boys tend to lag behind girls by a few months. Therefore it's probably a waste of time to push toilet training aggressively before age two since most kids don't have the building blocks to be successful.

WAYS TO GIVE YOUR TODDLER A BOOST

Eighteen-month-olds are so hands-on. They love anything tactile. Let them be messy and play with water, playdough, and sand. Let them use finger paints. They could build little towers of blocks and knock them down all day. Get them outside with a bucket, shovel, and a pile of dirt, and step back. If it's cold and rainy, get some rain gear on and go puddle stomping. If you are a clean freak and find yourself hovering to prevent a mess (I don't have a clean bone in my body and I *still* struggle with this), you might have to step a bit out of your comfort zone and give your child some space.

Your toddler's improved fine motor and spatial skills make puzzles an excellent activity. She'll love wooden puzzles with big, chunky pieces or little knobs to grab. She'll have fun with those shape sorters where you insert different blocks in the right holes. We had a secondhand bin of big wooden letters that our kids loved playing with, and it eventually helped them learn their alphabet.

I've said a lot about the importance of talking to your kids and reading books. You might notice that your eighteen-month-old is finally ready to "read" books with you rather than flip through the pages as quickly as possible or just play in the room while you read to her. Quick refresher on how to do so—animated and repetitive, with lots of intonation: "Where's the little blue truck? Do you see the little blue truck? There it is! There's the little blue truck!" Silly and repetitive, I know, but effective. This is where learning really takes off, and it's the perfect reason to make weekly trips to the library for a fresh stack of stories.

I know I've already preached about keeping your toddler away from screens as much as possible, but you're probably seeing now that she has quite a knack for electronics. She might be able to do things like unlock your phone or open picture albums on your tablet. And maybe you're aware of a bunch of learning apps. But still try to view those screens as an occasional distraction for plane trips or car meltdowns rather than a part of her daily routine. Remember that she learns from you most of all! Time with a screen means fewer interactions with you.

Remember at the start of this chapter when I noted how observant your child is? Well, she's also watching what you say and how you react to everything. She'll repeat bad words. She notices how you react when someone cuts you off in the car. She notices how you interact with people you pass on the sidewalk and cashiers at stores. When you argue with your partner, she notices the different tone of your voice and that your face looks angry. So be perfect always. Just kidding. Do be aware of what you do and say around your toddler, but don't be too stressed out by this—be excited that you have so much influence on your kid's values and character.

FAQS

Okay, I remember that we're supposed to ignore the tantrums, and that works pretty well at home. But what about when we're at the grocery store?

Tough one. Honestly, this is all about damage control. If possible, you scoop up your little one and get outside or into a bathroom. If you're by yourself with a cart full of groceries, you swoop in with a full-body pressure hug (pressure is just calming) and find something in the store to get *really* excited about within five seconds. If that doesn't work, you strap her into the cart to keep her safe, grab the essentials from your list, and move on. Survive to parent another day.

Our toddler is painfully shy. She won't look at anyone besides us, and she gets nervous in any new environment. Is that okay?

It's definitely okay. I think parents tend to stress out a little bit if their kid is the type that clings to their leg or buries her face in their lap around other people, especially when it's friends or family. Your kid is amazing and full of life, and you want the people you care about to see that too. My kids have always been shy, and when we take them to their pediatrician, I find myself bribing them with cash, prizes, and increased fatherly love to talk and make eye contact. It never works.

I'm sure you've seen those toddlers who will just walk up to other kids on the playground with a smile and start chattering away. One personality is not better than the other. Remember, at this age she looks to you for guidance and support, so that bond is the most important thing. She has years to get more comfortable with other people and with being away from you. Will she be the one crying with a death grip around your neck on the first day of kindergarten? Maybe, who knows? But kids are adaptable, and she'll do just fine.

Does my kid need a vitamin? If so, what kind should I give?

Probably not. If your toddler is eating a variety of healthy foods, she'll get all the vitamins and minerals she needs despite any ups and downs. There are just a few situations where a multivitamin can be a good idea:

1. Your child, despite your best intentions, does not reliably get green and orange veggies throughout the week. A multivitamin won't replace the fiber, but it will help fill in the gaps.

2. Your child gets less than eight ounces of milk a day. Cheese and yogurt can give her the calcium she needs, but a vitamin D supplement (part of any multivitamin) is a good idea.

3. Your child has a diet low in iron. As we talked about earlier, she needs that iron to make new blood. Kids get iron from meat, obviously—even turkey and chicken. There is also a good amount in most cereals, beans, peas, lentils, and eggs. Finally, dark green leafy veggies and dried fruits such as apricots, peaches, prunes, and raisins are a surprisingly decent source. If you're concerned, talk to your doctor or find a multivitamin that has iron in it (not all of them do).

There are a few different types of multivitamins available. Before they have molars, kids do best with a liquid vitamin. Most kids have molars by eighteen months, so children's chewable tablet vitamins are the best choice. Gummy vitamins are all the rage now, but dentists don't like them because they are basically fruit snacks that stick in the teeth and cause cavities. (It's also pretty hard to convince most toddlers that they aren't candy, which becomes dangerous if they somehow get ahold of the bottle.)

Do we have to get rid of the pacifier/binky/boo-boo/ Mr. Binkleton now? Our kid's pretty attached to it.

Not necessarily. What you want to avoid at this age is using the pacifier too much during the day. That will affect how often your child talks and how she pronounces words. So while it might be a quick fix for her frustrations, it's hindering the permanent fix—communicating what she's feeling. Also, the more often the pacifier is in her mouth, the more it could affect her teeth. It can cause an overbite where the top front teeth come down in front of the lower teeth.

I think it's perfectly fine at this age if she uses the pacifier at night, during naps, and for "special occasions" like airplanes and road trips. Your pediatrician and dentist can help you tell whether it's affecting her teeth. Some kids just suck on it to fall asleep, and other kids suck really hard all night—they're more likely to develop an overbite. If it's not affecting the teeth and is limited to sleeping times, it's probably fine up until age three.

Two Years

Two-year-olds are obsessed! They often come into the exam room with chubby fistfuls of trains smeared with a paste of crumbled crackers and sweat. Your two-year-old might also be obsessed with cars, construction, animals, dinosaurs, kitchenware, or princesses. And he'll keep you on your toes. As a parent you know that the "terrible twos" started a long time ago, but it's about to go to the next level. One minute he'll be counting to ten like a four-year-old, and the next he'll be convulsing on the floor because he dropped a fruit snack into the heater vent. Let's explore this wonderful world.

WHAT YOUR TODDLER SHOULD BE DOING NOW

For the last year or so I've been telling you to be patient with language, that it takes a long time to develop. Now language should be taking off. Your child should be saying around fifty words and starting to put two words together, like "Mommy help" or "Daddy home." It's not as important that the words are super clear. We're hoping to understand about half of what he says. Some two-year-olds spout off shockingly clear full sentences and some are well below fifty words. As always, whether your child is progressing is more important than where he's at with his speech.

Physically, your child should be zipping around the playground pretty well now. He should run and not fall as often as he used to. He should coil up his body as if he's going for the world record high jump and then get one millimeter of air. He should be able to kick a ball, and he should be fairly comfortable going up and down stairs.

Your toddler should be a pro with his fork and spoon by now. He should be coordinated enough to stack about six blocks and be even better at destroying them. He should be improving at coloring too—able to move a crayon *all around* your walls instead of just side to side.

Your child should be doing some imaginative play now, maybe pretending to cook just like you or flying an airplane on an adventure around the living room. Most of that play will still be by himself. Two-year-olds are checking other kids out but still prefer parallel play.

You should expect your toddler to have a short fuse. Tantrums and meltdowns can come out of nowhere, and it can be a Herculean task just getting into the car or going shopping. Your two-year-old gets some really intense feelings, but he doesn't yet have the impulse control to handle them. He's also probably into pushing limits. Tell yourself (again and again and again) that this is *good*. It's how he figures out boundaries.

DISCIPLINE—FINALLY, STUFF THAT WORKS!

Up until now, we've talked about how your available discipline tools haven't really kept pace with your child's behavior. Fortunately, his brain has finally developed enough to understand consequences, so you're about to make a comeback. Time-outs and positive reinforcement are lean, mean, and ready to give you the upper hand in molding your little citizen of the world. As with sleep training, discipline is a personal choice. There are many ways to do it, and you should decide what works best for your family, but I want to focus on some simple techniques that work.

TIME-OUTS

A time-out is a way of withdrawing attention to try to eliminate a behavior you don't want. It forces your toddler to sit alone without any toys or interactions for a brief period of time so that he'll learn what's okay and what's not okay. Setting up a good time-out system takes time, patience, and organization. It's an investment, just like sleep training. It's actually more painful (for you) than just caving in to bad behavior in the short run, but it will make your household less stressful in the long run. Here are some simple steps:

1. DECIDE WHAT BEHAVIORS DESERVE TIME-OUTS. You know your child best, but here are some things that would be reasonable to address with time-outs for a two-year-old:

    - Hitting, biting, pushing, or not being gentle with a newborn sibling
    - Touching something dangerous you've warned him about many times, such as an outlet
    - Not coming to you when you've called him many times, whether it's to get in the car or brush teeth
    - Throwing food or toys
    - Putting something in his mouth/nose/ear that he shouldn't

    Here are some things that don't translate so well to time-outs at this age:

- Most tantrums or meltdowns. If it's over something such as getting the red cup instead of the yellow one or not being able to watch *Frozen* for the thirty-fifth time, stick with being firm and ignoring it. *But*, if he's frustrated by something he's struggling with, such as fitting a puzzle piece, acknowledge that he's upset and move in to help him.

- Acting boisterous or yelling. That's kind of where two-year-olds are at. It's always fine to ask him to take a break or use his "inside voice" (get used to that one), but it's tough to expect a lot of self-control at this age.

- Not finishing his vegetables or other food. You don't really want to go down that road.

- Anything remotely related to potty training!

2. GET EVERYONE ON THE SAME PAGE. This includes grandparents (good luck with that) and nannies. If your child is in daycare, find out what they discipline for and how they do it. It's confusing for kids when consequences are not the same. Also, I'm sure you realize by now that toddlers are master manipulators—if they know they can get away with something with Dad but not Mom, they'll take advantage of him every time.

3. WORK OUT THE LOGISTICS OF THE ACTUAL TIME-OUT. You need a boring place near the center of the action, such as a bottom step or a corner. His room is probably too fun. If you have multiple levels in your home, have a time-out spot on each floor. You need to be decisive and move quickly so his brain can connect the time-out to what he just did. If he doesn't go quickly on his own, pick him up and calmly take him there. No

yelling needed. This is *not* a teachable moment yet. Two minutes is perfect for now (one minute for every year of age)—that will seem like a really long time to him. Ignore him during the time-out (try not to talk to or even look at him), even if he's really upset.

4. DEBRIEF *AFTER* THE TIME-OUT IS OVER. *Think firm but loving!* Ask him why he got the time-out and then talk about what he's going to do next time. Keep it short and to the point. Give him a quick hug and move on. I *don't* think you need to force him to apologize to anyone he may have hurt—try modeling good behavior instead by checking in with the offended party empathetically.

5. THE COUNTDOWN. Once your toddler knows that you're for real, a countdown becomes quite effective. After several warnings to him to put your phone down, your eyes are wide and you say in your no-nonsense voice, "If you don't put that phone down like I asked by the count of three, then you're going to get a time-out—one . . . two . . . thank you for listening."

Simple, right? Five easy steps for a lifetime of good behavior. I'd love to just stop there, but honesty compels me to tell you about all of the things that will probably go wrong. Let's do some time-out troubleshooting:

1. "It seems like we're just warning him all day long because no one actually wants to go through with the time-out." This is a common problem, and your kid will test those limits constantly. Give one warning, at most, and then go straight to the time-out. Unpleasant, but your child will quickly learn that you mean business.

2. "He laughs at us or does something bad just so he can run over and give himself a time-out." It's all about your tone. You're being too nice and allowing it to be a game.

Remember that the time-out needs to be abrupt and wordless. It's *funny* when kids give themselves time-outs, and many parents have told me that they can't help laughing. But try to be strong. He's putting on a show to see your reaction—so either turn away or stare at him with no expression on your face and your arms crossed.

3. "He won't stay in the corner—he runs away every time we put him there." Come on, now. Use your size and patience advantage here. Wait patiently, catch him when he tries to run, and place him back down. Five times, ten times, whatever it takes. Even if he does that for the whole two-minute time-out, it's not a fun experience and he'll learn the lesson. One more option is to put him in a boring (and safe!) room without any toys, such as a laundry room, where you can close the door.

4. "I can't really give him a time-out in the car or the store and he knows it, so what can I do?" You have my sympathies on this one. This is really just another version of your kid having a tantrum in a public place. I think there are a couple of options, none of them perfect. First, the time-out can consist of you withholding your attention for two minutes. That's pretty unpleasant for a lot of kids. The next option, especially when outings are starting to become difficult in general, is giving your child something special upon entering the store. This should be something reserved for this occasion only. And then you can *take it away* for a time-out if your child is throwing all the mac and cheese boxes on the floor. What doesn't work is a *delayed* time-out, like later in the car or at home. Remember that your toddler, genius though he may be, still doesn't have that long of an attention span.

Some people feel that time-outs are too mean or out of style. But evidence from numerous studies, talking to lots of families, and my own experiences as a parent tell me that they work. One 2012 study[50] in particular looked at forty-one different studies comparing both positive and negative (such as time-outs) forms of discipline. Negative methods were associated with better compliance in *every one*. Kids appreciate knowing where the limits are, they just don't realize it. They do well with predictable consequences, and after age two they are able to change their behavior in response to those consequences. I've said this before, but I want to emphasize it—*be confident in your bond*! It's like steel, forged in the fires of tears, blowout diapers, and sleep deprivation. Dramatic, I know, but if you truly believe that bond will carry you through it all, you're able be a better parent.

POSITIVE REINFORCEMENT

We've talked about negative consequences, but know that positive reinforcement is also a useful tool. This is different from bribery. In bribery, you're confronted with a tough situation and give an incentive to resolve it on the spot ("If you eat two bites of dinner, I'll give you some Skittles"). But positive reinforcement is set up *before the problem occurs*. Let's look at a few key points:

BE VERY SPECIFIC. It does *not* work to say, "If you're good this morning, you can watch *Curious George*." You need to be concrete. Focus on one frustrating behavior that you want to eliminate. Perhaps your child has been fighting getting strapped into the car seat lately. Before you leave the house, show your child that you are putting a favorite small toy in your pocket and explain what's about to happen: "We're going to go get in the car now. I'm bringing Spiderman with me. If you cooperate and get right into your car seat without a struggle, then you can have Spiderman in the car! Does that sound good?"

MAKE IT EASY. Set a low bar for your child at first. Maybe he's screaming a lot lately just for kicks. Tell him, "Your screaming hurts Daddy's ears. How about this? If you don't scream for five minutes, you can look at some pictures on Daddy's phone. Does that sound good?" Five minutes is easy, but you want him to succeed. Your little one is smart. Once he realizes that he has the power to get things through good behavior, he'll be more inclined to do it again next time.

USE APPROPRIATE REWARDS. In general, keep things small. Experiences, such as looking at pictures or listening to a favorite song, are ideal. Try to stay away from food for the most part. An exception is allowing kids to get a small amount of dessert after eating vegetables or other healthy foods (agreed to ahead of time). Set the bar very low—for example, we'd offer our kids a single chocolate chip if they'd eat their entire serving of veggies.

Sticker or star charts are a great way to work toward a bigger reward. Take a piece of construction paper and write the grand prize at the bottom, maybe a small toy, a trip to the pool, or a new book. Then draw five blank squares and you're set. Remember to be very specific about the ways he can earn his stickers.

I find switching to a positive reinforcement strategy is especially helpful when it seems like most of your interactions with your child are negative throughout the day (pretty common for two- and three-year-olds!). It's also crucial for kids with oppositional behavior, who can dig in and actually get energized by negative consequences.

POTTY TRAINING: LESS IS MORE

At eighteen months we talked about laying the groundwork for potty training: talking about pee and poop and having a few potties around to get comfortable with. At two there's more you can do, but don't get too excited! He's still going to use that potty when *he's* ready.

You can make good use of the positive reinforcement techniques discussed on page 164. The key is setting the bar low and taking very small steps. At first you might tell your child that he gets a sticker for telling you when he has gone pee or poop. You might then move on to reward sitting on the potty with his diaper on. When he's comfortable with that, you might raise the bar to sitting on the potty without a diaper. Eventually you can reward him if he does a little something on the potty. At all stages, use motivating language that helps him feel more confident, such as "It must feel nice not to be wet!" or "You're getting so big now!" If he seems stressed out at any point, just step back and relax for a while—don't bring it up as often and don't push it. And realize that progress is unlikely during times of change such as moving, starting daycare, or the birth of another child.

As I mentioned previously, never even *think* about punishing him or showing displeasure if he fails. He will fail a *lot*. He'll be kind of into the potty for a week and you'll think you're almost there—diaper freedom forever! You're *not* almost there, because for the next two months he'll decide that he has absolutely no interest in any of it. During this time, you could offer a reward that he would sell his soul for, but that doesn't mean he'll poop for it. When he's not into it, your job is to act like you don't really care. Casually bring it up every now and then to test the waters, but don't push. And remember to play it cool. Be excited when he takes a new step in training but don't go overboard. A lot of parents hoot and holler like they just won the lottery and that can weird kids out a bit.

At some point your child will decide he wants to pee on the potty and start to do it pretty consistently. This is a good time to start using pull-up diapers because they are quick to pull off and on and get him ready for underwear. And poop is its own thing, so don't be surprised if he's peeing in the potty like a champ for months but still creeping off behind the couch to poop in his diaper. Once he seems comfortable with both, you're ready for the big weekend, where you put him in those big boy undies he picked out and spend lots of time at home. Do fun things to keep him distracted and gently ask him if he has to go pee or poop every now and then. Accidents are no big deal. If you do have to go out, resist the temptation to throw him in a diaper for convenience. Bring a change of clothes and always know where the closest potty is. Lots of kids will still need a diaper at night for a few more months or even years, so that's totally normal. But you did it! Now get some good wine, make a bonfire with all your leftover diapers, and celebrate.

WAYS TO GIVE YOUR TODDLER A BOOST

Be okay with messes! Good structure and rules are crucial for your two-year-old, but healthy exploration involves a little mess. I've been at friends' houses where the parents follow their toddler around as if he's romping through a china shop. They instantly tidy up anything the child disturbs and give a lot of words of warning as he explores: "Careful, honey . . . Oh! . . . That's Mommy's crystal, honey . . . We've never used it but it's Waterford, honey . . . Can you say Waw-ter-ferd?" Create a lot of child-friendly spaces in your house, and then try to give him some freedom. Plus, what better way to spend your alone time after your little whirlwind goes to bed than cleaning?

Remember how I said that socialization wasn't super important before? That starts to change now. Your child should go from parallel play at age two to interactive play by three. To make this happen, he needs some exposure to other kids during the next year. Figuring out the rules of the playground requires contact with a lot of different kids. Playgrounds and indoor play places are great options. Maybe you've already started playdates with other kids, but if not, this is a good time to do so.

Most two-year-olds get really excited by books, and they can get a lot more out of them than they could six months ago. They can follow a story and start to understand some of the characters' emotions. Make reading a part of your bedtime routine every night. Even though two-year-olds would have you read their favorite book every night for months, make lots of trips to the library to keep things fresh (reading *Goodnight Moon* one hundred times might make you insane). If you want to spoil your child with gifts, get him books.

You can also help your child by starting to brush his teeth twice a day. Continue using a small amount of fluoride toothpaste, even if he swallows it. Also, now is a great time for his first visit to the dentist.

Finally, you can help your two-year-old—hold on, let me get back on my high horse here—by turning the TV off.

SCREEN TIME

At the two-year visit I really start to talk about screen time. Overall, I think that people work hard to limit screen time for their kids. I'm sympathetic to busy working parents who use the TV to occupy their children while they cook, shower, clean, or relax. Especially when there's a new sibling in the house or one parent is out of town. Household chaos is my everyday reality as well. There's a role for screens to help when you need to get things done. But a lot of kids get way too much.

Most parents stumble upon a dirty little secret somewhere along the way. They find that they can pop in (or "stream," or whatever else you techies are doing out there now) a Disney movie and get eighty minutes of peace and quiet. They can repeat the same one over and over again, *and* they get credit for giving their kids a special treat! So everyone feels good about it. I know this is judgy, but I don't think you *should* feel good about that. Maybe you should even feel a bit guilty. Your child is a ferocious learner, but you just paused his development for over an hour.

The American Academy of Pediatrics has some pretty strict screen time guidelines,[51] and with good reason. They recommend no screen time at all before eighteen months and then a limited amount of "high-quality" slow-paced programming over the next six months. From age two to five, they recommend less than one hour per day, recently reduced from two hours. They also advise no screen time during meals or within one hour of bedtime. I know that sounds strict, but a growing body of evidence shows us that getting too much screen time (particularly over two hours per day) can affect your kid's brain in a lot of negative ways:

- Total screen time is a risk factor for obesity.
- More screen time has been linked to less sleep,[52] even when it is not immediately before bed.
- Increased screen time is linked to delays in cognitive skills, motor skills, and language.[53]
- Two or more hours of screen time has been correlated with higher rates of attention problems in children.[54] Screens are very stimulating to our brains, and perhaps it's hard to match that stimulation in the "real world." Or perhaps the screen time changes how susceptible young brains are wired.
- Two or more hours of screen time per day has also been shown to cause more problems with behavior, controlling emotions, and interacting with peers.
- One recent study[55] also suggested that taking screens away from kids for several days improved their ability to recognize human emotion, implying that screens hurt kids' ability to recognize emotion—yikes!

One of the most common responses I get from parents when I ask about screen time is, "Well, the TV's on in the background but he doesn't really watch it—he's not that interested yet." I guess "secondhand TV" is better than staring at it for a long time, but I still worry about the effect it has on kids. Leaving the TV on in the background is quite common. A 2005 study of kids under age six found that 35 percent live in a household with the TV on all or most of the time, and that these children were less likely to be able to read compared with other kids.[56] Studies have also found that toddlers exposed to more background TV have a shorter attention span[57] and fewer interactions with their parents.[58] Plus, even if your two-year-old isn't that interested in TV right now, you can bet that he will be over the next few years! So try to get that TV turned off for at least some big chunks of the day—if you need background noise, maybe try music or a podcast instead.

Despite all my ranting, screens will play a big role in your child's future. It's okay for him to know how to navigate learning games or kids' websites on a tablet, for example. If he asks you a question, working together to find an answer on the internet is a great idea. How about TV? Can your child at least learn something from the limited amount of screen time that he gets?

A 2002 study[59] tried to answer that question by having kids between the ages of two and three perform a task after it was demonstrated either in person or on a screen. They all did great after the live demonstration, but only after two and a half were they able to understand the on-screen demonstration.

Most experts would agree that kids can start to do some real learning from quality programs such as *Sesame Street* or *Dora the Explorer* after age two and a half. (But remember, they *still* learn better from you at any age!) The new AAP screen time guidelines recommend that you watch *with* your child whenever possible until he's five years old. It's common sense that if you watch the program too and talk about some of the things that come up ("The Kratt brothers look kind of sad—why do you think they might be sad?"), that's probably a more stimulating experience for him.

FAQS

My friends all switched their toddlers to "big kid" beds at two. Is it time?

There's a strong sentiment out there that kids need to be moving to big kid beds at age two. I don't know where it came from, but I certainly don't agree. Cribs are the best! What could be better than a cage for your kid?! Seriously though, your toddler has associated his crib with calmness and sleep for a long time. It's safe and still plenty big. And two-year-olds are impulsive. In a crib, he doesn't have to fight the irresistible urge to go get the train across the room or go searching for you in the middle of the night. So my advice is to milk that crib for all it's worth. By three, most kids are getting a bit too tall and are thrilled by the prospect of a big boy or big girl bed.

There are a few exceptions. Some acrobatic kids start to climb out of their cribs as early as eighteen months, even when the mattress is at the lowest setting. If this becomes a habit, you're done and need to switch to a bed. (I've tried to think of other solutions, mostly involving Velcro, but to no avail . . .) Another decent reason to switch is if you have another baby on the way and don't want to buy a second crib for just a few months.

My friend told me that you can double a kid's height at two to figure out how tall he'll end up. Is that true?

Not at all. Parents are as obsessed with how tall their kids are going to be as they are with eye color. There's no magic way of knowing precisely, but genetics are powerful. The best way to estimate your child's height is by calculating something called the "mid-parental height." We basically add Mom and Dad's height together. But for a daughter we subtract five inches from Dad, and for a son we add five inches to Mom. Then we divide it by two. Most kids will fall within two inches of that height.

For example, let's say we're talking about a two-year-old boy whose mom is 5'4" and dad is 6'1". We would add five inches to the mom's height to make her 5'9". Then we average out 5'9" and 6'1" to 5'11". So the two-year-old is highly likely to end up within two inches of that. It may not be all that satisfying, but it's the best we've got.

My kid is the worst sharer of all time—probably below the 3rd percentile of sharing. What's wrong with him?

It is a universal experience of parenthood to be horrified when your two-year-old rips a toy away from another child, whether it's at the playground, story time, or even a friend's house. "Oh my God," you think to yourself, "Do they think I'm a crappy parent? Maybe I *am* a crappy parent." You then apologize to the kid's parents, pry the toy out of your child's fists, and try to get him to apologize. But he's screaming too hard because you took his hard-earned toy away.

But it's important to realize that it's *almost impossible* for toddlers to be good at sharing. Tovah Klein is a psychologist and author who specializes in toddler development. In an excellent article,[60] she concisely describes how toddlers don't have certain skills needed for sharing, including a sense of the feelings of others, a sense of time and patience, and the ability to override impulses. At ages three and four he will be more interested in making friends, which will help him to consider other kids' feelings and the effect sharing could have on those feelings. Klein points out that a common technique we parents use to foster sharing is taking turns, but younger toddlers don't typically understand that. Any given moment is just now, and they *want* it. So it's best to use calm, gentle guidance and distraction when navigating these sandbox battles. And as kids get older, they need a wider berth to try to figure this out on their own.

I'm planning on my child earning an athletic scholarship to college and then becoming a professional athlete. Or at least an Olympian. Any advice?

That sounds like a pretty solid plan. But in all seriousness, I think involvement in sports and physical activities is great. Learning movements that help in sports is kind of like learning a language. It's really easy when you're young because your brain is so flexible but becomes tougher as you get older. Plus, sports teach kids to listen and work together.

Some sports just don't work out for two-year-olds, like basketball, softball, and golf (unless he's Tiger Woods). But if you're looking for a structured activity, a few sports are awesome for this age. Throughout my career, I've noticed that kids in gymnastics now have better strength and balance when I see them at four or five. It gives them flexibility for whatever sports they might choose in the future. Soccer works well too and is available to two-year-olds in most areas. That ball just sits there and waits for them to whack it. Soccer gives them coordination, a team experience, and a sense of spacing that translates well to many sports. Dance, martial arts, and swim classes are other great options. Whatever you choose, keep it fun so your child becomes confident with his body. And, even though you probably won't need it, you might still want to save a *little* money for college just in case the scholarship doesn't work out.

I water down my kid's juice (usually doing hand gestures to illustrate half an inch of juice in an eighteen-inch-tall cup), so is that okay?

Sure it's okay, and the sugar is less concentrated. But it's still sugar your kid doesn't need, and you're setting the precedent of flavored water. The goal is to raise kids who reach for (plain!) water when they're thirsty.

I have to tell you about my favorite marketing strategy of all time. Nowadays all the apple juice makers sell apple juice with 40 to 50 percent less sugar. Brilliant! This finally solves the juice sugar problem! And then you realize that they took their apple juice, diluted it in half with water, and charged you the same price. Pretty awesome.

My kid loves to look at pictures on my phone. Does that count as screen time?

That's a great question. While most of the studies don't distinguish between different types of screens, common sense tells me that it matters. Any kind of screen can distract your child and decrease interactions with you, but screens that flicker and change rapidly (such as video games and cartoons) probably have a bigger effect on his attention and sleep patterns. As your child gets older, he'll probably engage with a tablet for hours a day during school and for homework. He'll be learning while doing this and staring at a mostly static screen, so I wouldn't count that (or looking at pictures) as screen time as long as it's brief.

Three to Four Years

Three- and four-year-olds are the seniors of toddlerhood. The "terrible twos" magically end on your child's third birthday, and the next fifteen years will be cake. And if you believe that, I have some swampland down in Florida I'd love to sell you. But seriously, by age three your child's thinking and impulse control are finally starting to catch up with her emotions and physical abilities. Tantrums happen less often. Her imagination is going to explode as she realizes there's a lot more out in the world than herself. She's going to ask you "Why?" hundreds of times per day. When I see her for her checkup, we're usually having fun again. She's back up on the exam table by herself after being in your lap since nine months. Specific milestones are less important than before—we start to look ahead toward kindergarten and whether she is developing the tools to be successful there.

WHAT YOUR TODDLER SHOULD BE DOING NOW

Up until now I've been talking about how *slowly* speech changes. Not anymore. Your child should be a *way* better talker now than she was at age two. She should be able to say five- to six-word sentences and have a few hundred words in her repertoire. She should be able to ask questions and do a decent job of answering questions. She shouldn't get as frustrated over expressing what she wants. All of this is still more important than how clear her speech is. We're shooting for strangers to understand about 75 percent of what she says at age three. By age four we want to understand just about everything. She should also be better at getting tenses and pronouns right. Even at four, however, it's still okay to struggle mightily with isolated sounds like "r," "s," and "th."

Your senior toddler's days of "toddling" (stumbling around like a drunken sailor) should be long gone. She should be running around confidently without falling very much. She should be able to jump forward with both feet at the same time. Even the really cautious kids should be loosening up a bit on the playground. She should be able to climb stairs with one foot per step just like you do. She should be able to draw some rough circles (*rough!*) by three and maybe triangles and squares by four. She should be pretty good at playing with toys that have moving parts, like levers, buttons, and switches.

Some of your kiddo's biggest changes involve her social skills and emotions. At age two she was scoping out other kids, but now she should be interacting with them once she's comfortable. For some three-year-olds that might mean making a few buddies to run around with on every playground visit, while for others might look like only being comfortable enough to interact with relatives or family friends who they see a lot. She should play differently now, with lots of make believe and fantasy. She used to be obsessed with toys themselves, but now they should be props to act out stories. Emotionally, your child is finally starting to realize that other people have feelings too. She's more likely to show concern for you if you're hurt, or to show affection for a friend without prompting from you. Her own emotions get more complex as well. Up until now you've mostly seen happy/excited and sad/angry. Now it gets a little more subtle. She can be bored, disappointed, surprised, puzzled, curious, suspicious, and lonely.

SLEEP REDUX

There's always stuff to talk about with sleep. Most three-year-olds are sleeping pretty well, but some new issues can pop up. Kids are out of their cribs now, so they can roam freely. They can come find you and try to get in bed with you, because why not? Their imaginations are running wild, so shadows and dreams can make nighttime a scary place. But it's like an arms race—their expanding little minds allow us to use some new tools.

There are a few common problems at this age. First, a lot of kids would rather play than sleep. They want to watch *one more* show, eat *one more* snack, hear *one more* story, and they're prepared to whine to get these things. Then, once they're in bed, they can take a long time to settle down. They can lay there singing or talking and keeping themselves awake. They can get up to play with their toys. Or they can think of every excuse possible to get you back in there: "I'm thirsty!" or "I've gotta pee!"

When your kid does finally fall asleep, you're *still* not out of the woods. Just like grown-ups, kids are cycling in and out of deep sleep at night. During good times, they just settle themselves back down without ever really being conscious. But sometimes they get into a bad habit of wanting you to do the settling and soothing for them. Sometimes this starts with an illness, a nightmare, or a change at home such as a parent going out of town for a few days. Maybe you let them crawl into bed with you or you lie in their bed until they fall asleep. They inevitably like the new arrangement and want to keep it long after the stressful period is over.

Sleep solutions are *never* easy, but there are a few powerful tools you can use to make things a little less painful:

SLEEP HYGIENE. This is all the background stuff you set up in advance to maximize the chances of your child sleeping well. Her body likes things to be the same for sleeping every night—she just doesn't know it. She likes to go to bed around the same time and after the same routine. She likes calming things like baths, comfy jammies, reading books, and singing quiet songs. She *thinks* her brain likes TV, tablets, and phones before bed, but it doesn't. Don't be fooled that she sits calmly and watches a screen, because meanwhile her brain's getting pretty excited—and excited brains don't sleep well. Whatever you do, *don't put a TV in her bedroom*!

BEDROOM PREP. Her room should be mostly for sleep. If it's her super-fun play place too, that creates temptation at night. Have lots of books on hand, but try to keep most of her toys elsewhere. If you have space constraints, try to keep her toys in bins with snap-on lids that you can store out of sight each night. Darkness is your friend—blackout curtains are crucial for naps and when the sun sets after bedtime. A very dim nightlight is great for kids who get scared or who are trying to get up to use the potty on their own. If you live in an apartment or have other kids making a ruckus, a white noise machine or fan can be helpful.

NOT GIVING TOO MUCH ATTENTION. When she gets up and comes to find you the first time, of course you're going to comfort her and make sure everything is all right. Maybe she had a bad dream or she has a fever. You'll probably do the same thing the second and third times. But don't bring her into your bed! Do that soothing back in her room, in her bed. When you start to realize that you're getting played (when she starts to call for you or come to your room most nights), you need to start turning down the attention. Even if you are putting her back into her bed, realize that kisses, hugs, songs, and lying next to her for a while are big-time positive reinforcers. So when you get to this point, just hustle her back to her bed with a quick "goodnight" and a kiss on the forehead and then leave the room. No negotiations. If she comes back one minute later, do the same thing. Of course you're slathering her with love the rest of the day. And remember that the promise of a little treat in the morning for staying in bed can give you some momentum. Just like with infant sleep training, a little pain up front prevents a lot of pain in the long term.

BEDTIME PASS. The bedtime pass is my secret weapon. This strategy is meant to work with kids age three and older who are having a hard time staying in their beds by themselves, whether when trying to fall asleep or in the middle of the night. You just take a little index card and decorate it with your child using markers, stickers, sparkles, or whatever. You can even laminate it with some clear tape to make it last a bit longer. Your child gets to keep the pass right next to her bed or under her pillow and can use it once a night to get a quick visit from you (for any reason, but it needs to be in her room). Then you take the pass from her and that's it for the night. Several studies have proven it to be effective, such as a small one from 2007[61] in which three- to six-year-olds struggling with sleep were treated either with bedtime passes or nothing. Those who used a bedtime pass were sleeping significantly better within ten days. In my experience kids typically stop using the pass within a few weeks—just knowing they have it gives them a sense of control and makes them feel more secure at night.

HANG ON TO NAPS. Around age three, a lot of kids start to fight naps. There's too much going on that they don't want to miss. So here's what happens: she misses a string of naps and then crashes at night because she's so tired. You give it your best effort but notice that now, when she *does* fall asleep for a nap, she's up late at night. A lot of parents throw in the towel at this point. But stick with it! She'll get back to her old pattern. Most kids benefit from a nap until age four and a half or five. Even when she's refusing to sleep, insist on at least an hour of quiet time each day, which will let her (and you) recharge.

HOW TO PRAISE YOUR KID

One of my favorite books as a parent is *Brain Rules for Baby* by John Medina.[62] Medina is a molecular biologist who starts with the science of how young brains work and then applies it to everyday situations where you can help your child. We all want our kids to be successful, and Medina identifies *effort* as the most important factor in success. And the key to raising kids who give a lot of effort is in how you praise them. It's natural to praise your kid for being smart, talented, or athletic—you're proud of her! But she doesn't have any control over her natural abilities. So she'll feel like her mistakes are failures outside of her control. She might be more concerned with looking smart rather than learning.

Medina describes a different "growth mindset" you can give your kid by praising her *effort*. Instead of saying, "You're so smart! I can't believe you figured out that sixty-piece puzzle!" say, "Wow, great job! You must have worked so hard to finish that!" These kids learn they can control their effort, and research has shown that they achieve more in school and even as adults. Medina specifically mentions some interesting work by researcher Carol Dweck. She found that kids praised for effort regularly finished 50 to 60 percent more difficult math problems than kids of similar ability who were praised for their intelligence. Praising effort doesn't come naturally, at least for me, so this is something I think about every day when I interact with my kids.

SOME THOUGHTS ON PRESCHOOL

In kindergarten your child will most likely have to be away from you for a full day. She'll have to sit still and know how to take turns and follow directions. She'll have to share and get along with twenty-five or so other kids, even if she's naturally shy. She'll have to be independent but able to ask for help as well. She'll need to be able to hold a pencil and write her name. She should have some strong building blocks for reading, like knowing her letters and even how some of them sound together. Maybe most importantly, she needs to be excited about learning new things.

This might seem kind of hard to envision for your three-year-old right now, but she'll get there. To be clear, your child does not *need* preschool to be successful in kindergarten, but I sure think it helps. It's not really about learning concrete things—she still does most of that with you at home. In preschool, she'll learn to socialize, which takes a lot of trial and error. She'll have access to toys and games that are different from what she has at home, and she'll unleash her imagination on them. She'll learn how to control her body. And the ubiquitous "circle time" is where it all comes together; she'll have to stop whatever fun activity she's doing and sit still. She'll have to focus on the teacher despite having a bunch of wiggleworms distracting her. She'll also have to learn how to do things as part of a group, like singing, as well as contribute when asked. Preschool is the start of her own little private life that's separate from you.

Preschool certainly does not need to be full time. Many parents start out with two or three half days per week at age three and then increase to four or five half days at age four. If your child is in day-care, many have preschool programs built in for ages three and four.

What should you look for in a preschool? Well, having gone through this process myself, I can say there's no way to avoid doing a lot of research. The price, location, hours, and availability of after-care (if needed) are the basics. I wouldn't get too hung up on the "philosophy" of the school (e.g., whether it's labeled Montessori or not). You want a place with a good blend of structured group time and lots of time to explore independently. I think a visit during regular hours (even more than just an open house) is crucial. The physical classroom should look *busy*. Remember that three- and four-year-olds have explosive imaginations that need lots of props. You want to see an art area, a dress-up area, a light table, a picture book area, puzzles, blocks, toys, animals, and outdoor space. Kids should be having fun and acting silly, but the teacher should have control of the classroom. A "firm but loving" approach works as well at school as it does in your home.

Class sizes vary a lot. Limits for state-funded preschool programs range from sixteen to twenty-four students. Private preschools can do whatever they want. The National Institute for Early Education Research has concluded that preschool class sizes of fifteen or smaller can improve learning outcomes. I think having two teachers (or a teacher and parents at a co-op) in the classroom is important as well. There will be plenty of times when one teacher is tied up with a behavioral or bathroom issue, so having a second adult keeps things running smoothly.

Of course, you can get your child ready for elementary school without preschool, but it takes more careful planning. She'll need some activities with structure, like library story time, gymnastics, or swimming lessons. She'll need plenty of unstructured time to figure things out with other kids, both on play dates with friends and in more chaotic environments like playgrounds.

While the benefits of preschool are easy to imagine, it's nice to reinforce that with some research. The Abecedarian Project was a fascinating study started over forty years ago in North Carolina.[63] They separated at-risk infants into two groups, one that received high-quality childcare and preschool and one that did not get any extra help prior to kindergarten. The researchers then followed the kids until they were thirty and found that the group with better early childhood education achieved more throughout their lives (including a higher IQ).

This study is old and not perfect—your child might not be "at risk" and might do just fine with or without preschool. But what I take away from it is that little brains are very flexible, and we have the ability to affect the course of our kids' lives by what we do before age five. That's really exciting, and I hope that someday all kids get access to high-quality early education without having to be enrolled in a study.

WAYS TO GIVE YOUR TODDLER A BOOST

The student has become the teacher! Up until now you've been your child's tour guide through life. You've taken her outside and taught her what everything is. You've shown her how to play with blocks and how to identify a bunch of animals. You've ushered her around the playground and encouraged her to slide and swing. Now you've got to get out of the way.

FLOOR TIME

We all have agendas for our kids and are eager to teach them more than we have time for. Sometimes it's nice to set that agenda aside and let your kid hop into the driver's seat. Floor time is a simple but powerful concept that can help busy parents like you give your kid some control and see where her mind goes. Dr. Stanley Greenspan was a child psychiatrist who developed the concept over forty years ago for kids with autism. But in its simple form it can be a secret weapon for all parents. Try to set aside fifteen to thirty minutes several times per week where you are literally down on the floor with your child following her lead. She's the boss. When it's silly or awkward, resist the urge to redirect her. You *can* encourage, facilitate, and make sound effects. This time should be protected, never taken away as punishment or disrupted by a phone. This time means the world to her, and secretly you'll know that it's a fantastic way to build her brain.

Floor time is also a great way to deal with three- and four-year-olds who are acting up. Sometimes she's caught in a cycle of seeking negative attention from you, and your frustration only makes it worse. Floor time gives her the attention she craves in a healthier way.

Your child is learning all the time, but what about more direct teaching at this age? Is that a good idea, or will it crush her love of learning? This can be a touchy subject, but let's tackle it reasonably. For instance, it's great to build a foundation for kids to be strong early readers. To do this she needs to be able to identify upper- and lowercase letters and the sounds they make. But don't make flashcards—it has to be fun. So maybe when you're reading a book you have her try to find all the "As." Or sing a song she likes and say all the "Ts" so hard that you're almost spitting.

It's great to get kids comfortable with numbers too, but you need to make counting visual, like by moving forward spaces while playing a board game, or seeing that three blocks is the same as two blocks plus one more block. Stories are also great for teaching some math. My kids were always thrilled to hear stories about "doing bad things." For example, "Mama made five cookies and set them out to cool. But then your brother snuck into the kitchen and took two of them! How many were left? What if you caught him and made him put one back—now how many are there?"

Some people say, "Kids learn this stuff in kindergarten anyway, so why do it earlier? They should just be having fun." Of course kids should be having fun. There's a lot of time in the day, though, and if you mix some learning in with the fun, I think it puts your child at an advantage. Being able to read lets her explore things she's interested in, even when you can't sit with her. Being good with numbers will help her to understand time and money, and to play many different games. Some kids might understand this stuff at age four and some might not get it until six or seven, but I don't think it's pushy to work on it through play.

Can teaching go too far? Absolutely. With some coaxing and bribing you might be able to get your kid to sit for fifteen minutes and work on a list of letters or numbers. But I'd say there's a cost to that—*excitement* about learning is one of the most important and fragile things to cultivate in your kid over the next few years. Also, kids can memorize and mimic pretty well at this age, but they're not really learning when they do that. Resist the urge to teach your child "party tricks," like memorizing simple math, sports trivia, or parts of books. (It's entirely possible that I tried to teach my son all the state capitals when he was three.)

For physical skills, this is a great time to start the whole bike-riding process. (Note that I do *not* recommend my own father's method, which involved setting me on my Schwinn banana seat at the top of an incline with a push and a "good luck." Even though it *was* quite effective. Fear really hones the senses.) Bicycling increases strength and coordination and gives your kid a great way to exercise and explore for the rest of her childhood. I'll bet when you were little you went through the time-honored tradition of training wheels. They're still around, of course, but there's a new kid on the block—balance bikes. You've seen these before: they're mini bikes made of metal or wood without any pedals at all. Europeans have been using them for a long time, and I think they were right on this one. Kids can start riding them around age two or three, just walking with the bike at first but then running and gliding as they get more comfortable. It gives them a better sense of balance than the training wheels, and most kids are able to start working on the big kid bike without training wheels around age four. And don't forget the occasional baseball card in the spokes to make the bike sound like a motorcycle—that's just plain cool.

BACK-SAVING BIKE BAR

I'm not really into gadgets, except when they save my lower back from pain and destruction. My neighbor gave me a bar with a nice padded handle that attaches to the seat column of a big kid bike and extends up a few feet. This has prevented me from having to sprint while bending at ninety degrees to grip the back of the seat as my child careens toward the only pole in a huge parking lot. It's a nice option, especially if you are tall, inflexible, and aging.

FAQS

My child started stuttering a few weeks ago. Will it go away? Do we need speech therapy?

Stuttering is pretty common between age two and five, especially in boys. It can start abruptly and be really impressive—I once sat quietly for a full minute while a three-year-old patient tried to get through the word "stethoscope." Stuttering happens more when the child is excited, anxious, or tired. Fortunately, there's little cause for concern. It almost always resolves within a few months and is usually not associated with other developmental problems. No one knows for sure why it happens, but it might be a sign of your child learning tons of new words at once without being great at using them in sentences yet. Or it might mean that her thoughts are racing ahead of her words, and stuttering gives her words a chance to catch up. In my experience, most stutterers at this age are really verbal kids.

These kids are usually happily oblivious to their stuttering, and you should keep it that way. Never try to change it or coach them through it—if they become self-conscious, it will only get worse. Just listen patiently as they work it out. Serious stuttering after age six is different. It's less likely to go away and can be a barrier to learning as well as a source of social embarrassment. In that case, the child should be evaluated for speech therapy.

My kid is kind of pigeon-toed and she sits with her legs in a "W." My friend told me this could get worse when she's older and that I should tell her to sit "crisscross applesauce" style. Thoughts on this?

Most little kids are kind of pigeon-toed. Their thigh bones (femurs) are naturally rotated in a little where they attach to the hips. Some kids are turned in quite a lot, and we call this "femoral anteversion." These kids are most comfortable sitting with their legs splayed out to the sides in a "W." A long time ago doctors occasionally put kids in braces or splints to try to fix the problem. Only ten years ago, I was trained to encourage kids to sit with their legs crossed to help fix it.

Now we know that almost all of these kids do fine no matter what interventions are made. Their femurs tend to rotate out more after age five and are usually normal by ten. Some of these kids might trip over their feet a bit more than others when they really get moving, but it shouldn't prevent them from keeping up with other kids. And, for these children, sitting crisscross style is like you trying to sit in a W—uncomfortable. So don't worry about it.

I think my three-year-old had a seizure! When I took away her snack she got really upset, stopped breathing, fell back onto the carpet, and shook for almost ten seconds before she was "with it" again. What should I do?

Anything that looks like a seizure is scary! Fortunately this is just a breath-holding spell, and it's fairly common for toddlers and preschoolers. Some kids are more prone to them than others. It usually occurs when they're very upset, surprised, or scared. It's *not* intentional. They can get a bit purple in the face and pass out. When they pass out they can twitch or shake for a few seconds, and then they are immediately alert. They will always breathe at that point. The only risk is hitting their heads when they pass out. Seizures tend to happen at more random times, involve more sustained shaking, and leave kids dazed for a few hours afterward.

There's a trick that I like to recommend for parents whose kids do this a lot. When you see her getting really upset and you don't hear those breaths anymore, blow a quick blast of air right into her face. This usually triggers her to start breathing again.

My kid makes *so much* earwax. She's like a candle factory. Almost every day I'm having to clean her ears. Is that normal?

I hear this question a *lot* for little kids. Earwax is kind of like sweat—some people make a lot and some make a little. But I usually reassure parents that it's *good* if you see a lot of wax. Seeing it means that, even if she produces a lot, her ears are pushing it to the outside of her ear canals and away from her ear drums. It's always fine to grab the wax you can see by twirling a cotton swab or using a wet washcloth around a finger. But never put the swab *into* the ear canal—you'll get some out but you'll push some in toward the ear drum as well. This can create impacted plugs of wax that affect your child's hearing. I often have to get that stuff out in the office.

There are some kids who legitimately make tons of wax that blocks up their ear canal every few months. There is a nice over-the-counter product called Debrox for such occasions—these carbamide peroxide drops dissolve the wax. You put in five drops, let it sit for ten to fifteen minutes, and then flush it out with some warm water using a bulb syringe. Make sure that you do it twice a day for three days to get everything out. Some kids need this done every two or three months. The package says it's safe for kids over twelve, but I think it's fine down to age three or four.

My daughter is going to turn five just a few months before kindergarten starts. Do you think I should hold her back another year?

This is a question I get asked a lot and it's a really tough one to answer. For most school districts, the cutoff for starting kindergarten is turning five by September 1 (give or take a month). Certainly there has a been a trend over the past decade to hold kids, especially boys, back a year even if they turn five in the months leading up to the deadline. Parents have a variety of reasons for doing this. Some don't want their kid to be the youngest and smallest in the class—at age five, being ten months younger than your classmates is a big difference (although the difference becomes less significant the older they get). Others frankly feel that their kid will be more competitive academically and athletically if they are one of the oldest in the class. Some parents are concerned that their child is too shy or immature. And there is a perception, possibly true, that boys can take longer to be behaviorally and emotionally ready for kindergarten.

There is really no right answer for every family, but I would consider a few things. First, think hard about the next year—which choice would lead to the most growth in your child? A third year of preschool where she is the oldest could get boring, while kindergarten might have a pretty steep learning curve at first but still be very stimulating for her. Remember, the first few months of kindergarten are for ironing out the kinks—she's not expected to come in knowing how to perform perfectly. Also, experienced preschool teachers have worked with hundreds of kids. I would give a lot of weight to their opinions about your child's readiness. Finally, sports are important and I hope they're a big part of your child's life, but I don't think they should play any role in deciding when to start kindergarten.

All that being said, I think there *are* some good reasons to hold off on starting kindergarten. If your child has significant problems with aggression, frequent meltdowns, or anxiety beyond normal shyness, discuss it with your pediatrician. Also, you might want to think about waiting a year if your child has not shown much improvement with learning letters and numbers, or is more likely to get extremely frustrated by "failure" than motivated to push through when facing a challenge.

My three-year-old daughter is "playing with herself" all the time—is this normal? Should I put an end to it?

This is a common concern, actually. Boys and girls touch and play with their genitals just like they do with other parts of their body, like their ears when they're younger. Boys especially can get pretty rough and tug on their penises in a way that looks painful (don't worry—he won't hurt himself). Your child may do this for fun or to soothe herself when she's tired or nervous. It's completely normal, so I wouldn't put an end to it. We want kids to have a positive view of their bodies and not to be ashamed of them. However, I do think that around age three is a reasonable time to make a distinction between what is okay in private and what is okay in public. So calmly tell your child that touching her genitals is something for home and gently remind her if she forgets while you're out.

Our four-year-old daughter has an imaginary friend named Lulu who lives in our house's HVAC system and shoots glitter from her eyes. Should we just start counseling now or wait until kindergarten?

The pendulum has swung back and forth with imaginary friends. Back in the day (just a few decades ago) leading pediatricians and psychologists thought imaginary friends indicated a void in the child's life. They thought these kids were troubled introverts who struggled with real relationships. And most people just thought those kids were kind of weird. But over the past two decades, new research has turned the conventional wisdom on its head. Children with imaginary friends have been found to have better communication skills[64] and more creativity[65] than other kids. And, even though imaginary friends peak between ages three and five and are usually gone by nine, these benefits seem to last through adulthood! Kids with imaginary friends have basically found an extra way to work out their creativity and play muscles. So no counseling necessary—at least for this.

Cases

Your child is going to get sick and injured. It will happen at home, or in daycare, or on a plane. It will happen in the middle of the night or in the middle of the day. It might come on slowly or hit suddenly. When it happens, you will need to make some decisions. Do you need to take your child to the doctor? What can you do to make him feel better? What red flags should you look for? You probably didn't go to medical school, and even if you did, that part of your brain tends to malfunction when it's *your* kid. So you'll rely on talking to family and friends to see what they think. You might creep onto Google to get some answers and end up terrified (pretty much anything can be a sign of leukemia). Hopefully you're able to call your pediatrician's office any time you need to as well.

I want to give you one more resource that will help you deal with some of the more common things that come up. I always learned best from cases. I think a little story with people's names and symptoms makes it easier to remember the details of a particular disease. I'm guessing it will be the same for many of you. Illnesses don't happen in a vacuum. They happen in families with all kinds of stuff going on that can complicate the illness—where both parents work, for example, or when one parent is out of town for the week, or when Grandma and Grandpa are watching the kids. So these cases will be about families just like yours. Hopefully that will make it a bit more fun than WebMD, and maybe some of it will stick with you when you are confronted with a similar scenario in your life.

You can use this section in two ways. It could act as a reference when issues pop up, or you could spend a little time reading it beforehand so you're more confident when these illnesses surprise you.

THE BASICS

First let's set some illness ground rules:

- A fever is 100.4 degrees Fahrenheit or higher. Let's be clear about that. I often hear, "Well, my child runs low so I know that when he's at 99, he's got a fever." *Nope*. A fever starts at 100.4 for any child—then everyone is on the same page and we avoid confusion. And don't add a degree if you check under the arm or subtract a degree if it's hot outside or anything like that. Just keep it simple and trust the thermometer. If it's right under 100.4, check it every thirty minutes until you know it's not rising anymore.
- There is also some confusion about duration of fever. If it's Thursday, and your child's fever started on Tuesday, then he has had *two* days of fever, not three (even though he has had a fever on three separate days). That difference is important in deciding when your child should come in. Calculate days by how many twenty-four-hour periods have passed.
- Realize that terminology matters. For medical folks, the word *lethargic* is scary. That's a kid who's not doing well at all, who's limp and not interacting or making much eye contact with you. A kid who's truly lethargic needs to be seen right away. So think about whether your child is *truly* lethargic, or if he's just tired and clingy.

- Everyone's goal should be to avoid antibiotics whenever possible. Antibiotics are crucial when your child needs them. But they come with a price. The more your child uses them, the less effective they are, because bacteria are really good at developing resistance. Antibiotics can also cause allergic reactions and other rashes, and they kill off some of the good bacteria in your child's intestines. Parents impress me nowadays. Most of them know that antibiotics don't do anything for viruses, and it's pretty rare that they come in looking for a prescription. When your child does need antibiotics, remember to start her on probiotics right away and continue for a few days after the course of antibiotics is finished.

THE PLACEBO EFFECT

The placebo effect occurs when you use a treatment that (unknown to you) has no proven benefit but you still experience an improvement in symptoms. I think it's important to understand this phenomenon and how it relates to your child's health. Your brain is really powerful, and when it expects something to work, it's often going to trick you into believing that it *is* working. The placebo effect is *everywhere*. Eating chia seeds is good for you in the long run, but you might suddenly feel an energy boost a few minutes after you eat them because you are expecting them to work some health magic in your body. When you give your one-month-old some gripe water for colic, you'll probably feel like it's reducing her fussiness (it's not). When you rub some menthol ointment on your child's chest when she has a cold, you'll probably feel like she sleeps a bit better (she won't). These are not necessarily bad things—if the placebo is not harmful, feeling better about helping your child is great.

SPEAKING OF THE PLACEBO EFFECT . . .

Walk through the pharmacy aisle at your grocery store, and you'll see no shortage of medicines that promise to boost your child's immune system to ward off illness and help her fight off a cold. Echinacea, Airborne, cough syrups, high doses of vitamin C, elderberry, lemon balm, and plenty of others. You might think, *We did it! We cured the common cold! Yay!* Except we didn't, and none of these things has been shown to work at all, and there are a lot of people who want to make money off your desire to help your child. It's true that vitamin deficiencies can make children more prone to illness, but it's *not true* that extra doses of vitamins or nutrients can help fight off an illness. Most cold and cough medicines are not recommended until six years of age, and it's quite clear that they don't work anyway (see cough syrup on page 211). Throughout the different cases, we'll talk about what you *can* do to help your child when she's sick—just know that the answer is not usually going to be over-the-counter medicine.

I make use of the placebo effect as a doctor too. When I tell you to use a humidifier for your toddler's cold, maybe it will prevent snot from hardening in his nose, but helping you to *feel* that you're helping him is probably a bigger benefit. I have to keep in mind that if I start a medicine for your baby's bad reflux, you'll probably feel like it is helping even though studies show it doesn't. When I am treating someone with a medicine for depression, I'm counting on the placebo effect to help them start feeling better weeks before the medicine is at an adequate dose. Good studies, and many of the ones I reference in this book, are "placebo-controlled," which means that they compare the treatment they're studying with a placebo that looks the same. Then researchers can say with more confidence that a benefit is due to the treatment itself and not just the placebo effect.

But realize that people can take advantage of this placebo effect and your desire to find a solution. This is a good place to apply healthy cynicism. If you use expensive essential oils on your kid's tummy when he has a stomach virus, you're likely to believe that they helped him get better within a few days (when in reality, the virus has just run its course). If you cut gluten from your child's diet in an effort to improve her behavior problems, you're inclined to feel like she does a bit better even if her behavior is actually the same. A chiropractor might recommend weekly (and expensive) craniosacral therapy to treat your newborn's colic, and your investment will probably make you perceive that it's helping despite absolutely no good evidence that it does (again, any improvement may simply correlate to your child aging out of the colic stage). A medical provider at an urgent care might suggest treating your child's four-day cold virus with an antibiotic, and you might notice that he starts to get better a few days after that. But now if he truly needs antibiotics in the future they might not work as well.

In short, try to weigh the benefits against any potential "harm" before starting a course of action. You can also control your own "placebo effect" in two ways: by distinguishing good evidence from bad evidence, and by being consciously aware of how your brain wants to believe the results you're expecting.

COLD

Amelia is a four-month-old cutie pie with blue eyes and absurdly long lashes. She's never had so much as a runny nose. After months of searching, her mom found the perfect daycare in a little church basement, which made her feel comfortable returning to work part time. Amelia's first day was two days ago—only two days!—and she woke up last night with a snotty nose and a 101-degree fever. Could she really catch something that quickly? She had a rough night—she was up every hour crying and her breathing has been pretty snorty. She hasn't been quite as interested in feeding. She's not really coughing. Her eyes aren't goopy, and she doesn't have any rashes. Should her mom take her to the doctor? Can she still go to daycare, or does her mom need to call in sick?

Colds are miserable. And yes, she *can* catch something that quickly—incubation periods for most viruses are around one to seven days. The good thing about them is that infants and toddlers are great at fighting them off. The bad thing is that there is very little *you* can do to help that happen more quickly. You need to distinguish the annoying but normal features of a cold from the complications that can get your child into trouble.

WHAT'S NORMAL FOR A COLD?

- Fever with the cold that can last up to five days and often spikes at night.
- Runny nose and cough (which often starts a few days later) for up to a full two weeks.
- Trouble sleeping at night, mostly due to gagging on all that snot, which makes it hard to breathe.
- Eating less solid food, sometimes none, and drinking a little bit less than normal. Infants have to breathe through their nose while breast- or bottle-feeding, so it can be especially hard for them to eat and breathe at the same time.

- Being more clingy than normal and not wanting to play as much.
- Snot that's clear, white, yellow, green, brown—a nastier color does not mean that your child has a sinus infection.
- "Boogers" in the corners of her eyes or some thin white goop on her eyelashes, especially when she first wakes up.

WHEN SHOULD YOU WORRY?

- The fever lasts for more than five days.
- The fever goes away for more than twenty-four hours but then comes back again. Or if your child develops a fever after she's already been sick for more than two days. Either can mean that she's developing a bacterial infection.
- Her energy isn't improving after being sick for a week. Or her energy starts to improve for a day or two but then starts to get worse again.
- She has thick yellow goop in her eyes that has to be cleaned constantly, or the whites of her eyes are getting red.
- She's drinking less than half of her normal amount and starts to have significantly fewer wet diapers.

WHAT CAN YOU DO TO HELP?

Okay, it makes me a bit nervous to say this to you, but you deserve to know the truth. *Nothing helps your child's cold.* I think it's important to be comfortable with that as a parent. Your child is going to suffer through lots of colds and be kind of inconsolable, and you're not going to get much sleep during the worst of it. You should hold her a lot and work hard to keep her hydrated, and she will do just fine. That being said, sometimes when you're frustrated that you can't do more to help, it's good to have some things to work on. Just the act of *doing something* for her can help get you through a long night. So, after I just told you that you can't really help your child, let's go over some ways you can help your child.

SUCTION. The amount of snot your kid can produce will shock you, and it's the snot that makes sleeping and feeding difficult. You can at least get a little bit of it out by putting a few drops of saline in each nostril and sucking the mucus out with one of those rubber bulb syringes. You can also use a NoseFrida, which is a smart little apparatus through which you provide extra suction power with your mouth. Yes, it sounds gross, but it is effective. Note that suction becomes a tough sell after about nine months because your child will kick you in the throat if you come near her nostrils.

HUMIDIFIER. Tried and true, the humidifier is always a good idea during a cold, especially in the winter when the air is dry and your heater is running. Lungs and throats are happier when they're moist.

SUPER STEAMER. Steam is your friend. Bring your kid into a bathroom with the shower cranked up very hot, close the door, and hang out and play for ten to fifteen minutes before she goes to bed. That steam will loosen up the crud in her nose and it's quite satisfying to see some of it flow out.

ELEVATION. Get gravity on your side. Anything you can do to elevate your child's head relative to her feet will help with snot drainage at night. For infants you're usually limited to a modest wedge under the head of the crib mattress, but some older toddlers might do well with a couple of pillows.

WHAT HAPPENED WITH AMELIA?

Amelia's mom calls her pediatrician's office, and the triage nurse feels that she is okay being managed at home. Even though Amelia is miserable with all the mucus production, she's still breathing well and staying hydrated. The nurse advises Mom that Amelia will probably get a bit of a cough when things start to drain over the next few days. Her congestion and cough could last for ten to fourteen days, but she'll probably start to feel better in four or five. She tells Mom to call back if Amelia's fever lasts longer than five days or if she's drinking poorly. Amelia can't go back to daycare until her fever has been gone for twenty-four hours, but Mom is happy to stay home and snuggle with her.

A WORD ON SINUS INFECTIONS

Sinus infections are a common concern of parents when their children show cold symptoms, especially when the snot gets thick and yellow or green. But sinus infections are pretty rare in little kids. Sinuses are open spaces in the facial bones that are normally filled with air. The two biggest are under the eyes just inside the cheekbones (maxillary sinuses), and above the eyes in the lower middle part of the forehead (frontal sinuses). No doubt you've felt some pressure in these areas at some point with a bad head cold. Newborns barely have these spaces, and they slowly grow throughout childhood. It turns out that thick green snot isn't a good indicator of a sinus infection. And your three-year-old isn't likely to say, "Mommy, I'm experiencing some facial tenderness." So let's talk about clues that *can* mean your child does have a sinus infection:

- A cold that lasts more than ten days *without improvement*. It's common for a runny nose or cough to last for ten days, but your child's energy and appetite should be better and the cough and congestion should be less intense. The key here is a total lack of improvement.
- Your child's cold starts to get better and then gets worse again. Once viruses start to improve they should stay on that course. So if a fever goes away and then comes back a few days later, or cough and congestion are improving and then go downhill again, you should visit the doctor.
- Hard-hitting illness from the beginning. This means that your child gets a fever greater than 102.2 degrees F with a ton of thick nasal discharge for at least three straight days. Plenty of viruses cause a higher fever than that with different symptoms, so the key here is the abundance of thick snot.

ALLERGIC REACTION

"Oh boy, this is not good," thinks Mason's dad. Mason is a barrel-chested thirteen-month-old. His mom left an hour ago for her first "girls' night out" since Mason was born. Dad got some pad thai delivered for him and Mason to share—mild, of course (he's no fool). He remembers that Mason's doctor said anything was okay to eat after the twelve-month visit. Mason helped dad shove in the first bite of delicious noodles and shrimp covered in peanut sauce and thought it was pretty awesome. But a few minutes later, Mason started to cry and vomited—real vomiting, not just spit-up. Now as Dad is holding him he watches some hives appear on Mason's chest and thighs. Mason is really upset, but his lips aren't swollen and he seems to be breathing fine. What should Dad do? Take Mason to the emergency room? Call 911?

Allergic reactions are scary, especially when you're all alone. They can happen so suddenly, and everyone knows that they can get bad enough to affect your child's breathing. Food allergies are also quite common, and are mostly due to a few heavy hitters (see the list on page 202). Between six and eighteen months, kids are trying new foods all the time, so it can be tough to pinpoint the exact source. Sometimes it takes a few exposures to a food before kids get sensitized to it, which is even more confusing.

WHAT ARE THE SIGNS?

- Symptoms appearing within a few minutes to a couple hours after eating something.
- Hives scattered over your child's body. This is a puffy red rash raised up off the skin in weird patterns. They're itchy and usually warm to the touch. Most notably, they come and go and move around. Once they start, they can last for a few days.
- Vomiting shortly after eating followed by bad tummy pain. If it's an allergy, the lining of your child's stomach is probably angry and inflamed.
- Very concerning signs include lip swelling and difficulty talking, breathing, or swallowing. (These require emergency action!)

- Listen carefully to how your child talks about his symptoms: kids have interesting ways of describing things. He might complain of his tongue feeling itchy, something being stuck in his throat, or his tummy tingling.

WHAT IS *NOT* A SIGN?

- A mild red rash limited to the skin around their mouth and the diaper area after eating certain foods. This is typically a food sensitivity rather than a true allergy. This means that it is superficial and does not involve immunoglobulin E (IgE), a chemical in your body that sets off the inflammation in true allergies. The most common offenders are acidic foods such as tomatoes, citrus, melons, and sometimes even carrots. This reaction should diminish as your child gets older and can be treated with petroleum jelly and maybe a little swipe of hydrocortisone.
- An impressive spit-up right after eating *without* a lot of discomfort afterward. Sometimes kids just eat too much too fast.

WHAT CAN YOU DO TO HELP?

- Benadryl (diphenhydramine) should be one of the things at the ready in your medicine cabinet. If your child's symptoms are limited to hives or an upset stomach, you always have time to start with Benadryl at home. After the first few hours anaphylaxis is unlikely, but you might have to give Benadryl for a few days to treat the hives and itching.
- If your child's lips are swollen you should give a dose of Benadryl on your way to the emergency room. For any trouble breathing or swallowing, you should give Benadryl immediately after you've called 911.
- Regardless of the severity, you should call your doctor to discuss the situation. Your doctor may want to have some allergy testing done. Kids with certain allergies need an epinephrine shot (EpiPen) at home that can stop a severe reaction.

WHAT HAPPENED WITH MASON?

Since Mason doesn't have any trouble breathing or lip swelling, Dad has time to give him some Benadryl. A half hour later he seems more comfortable, and the hives are not as angry-looking. Mason falls asleep, and Dad calls the pediatrician's advice line. The nurse recommends repeating the Benadryl as needed throughout the night and coming in for an appointment the next day to talk about his probable peanut allergy.

ALLERGY FAST FACTS

- Eight foods cause 90 percent of allergies: milk, eggs, peanuts, tree nuts, soy, wheat, shellfish, and fish.
- The American Academy of Allergy, Asthma, and Immunology estimates that about 8 percent of children have a significant food allergy.[66]
- The CDC estimates[67] that the rate of food allergies in children increased by 50 percent between 1997 and 2011. That's a big jump! No one knows for sure why.
- Children with food allergies are two to four times more likely to have asthma, eczema, or environmental allergies.
- Many kids outgrow allergies to milk, eggs, soy, and wheat by the time they start kindergarten. Nut, shellfish, and fish allergies are often lifelong.[68]
- Your child can be tested for allergies with a blood test ordered by your pediatrician or skin testing performed by an allergist.

PINK EYE

Maisie is an eighteen-month-old who was born at thirty-two weeks. Her parents were told that she would be smaller than other kids and take quite a bit longer to hit her developmental milestones. She apparently didn't get the memo and has stormed her way up to the 75th percentile for height and weight. She's already putting two words together and can run circles around plenty of "full-termers." Yesterday, her mom took her to Dizzy Castle, an indoor play place that's a madhouse of tangled toddlers and their bodily fluids. Maisie had fun and especially enjoyed trying to lick every ball in the ball pit. This morning she woke up with her eyes nearly glued shut. Mom was able to get the gunk off with a warm rag, but every hour there's more thick yellow stuff sticking to her eyelashes. The white part of her left eye looks a little bit red. She doesn't have a fever and seems pretty happy. Is this the dreaded pink eye?

Pink eye (or conjunctivitis) is an infection of the tissue around your eye, and it's a stinker. I don't think any other single illness wreaks as much havoc on daycares, preschools, and parents' work schedules. It's not the most dangerous condition in the world, but it looks god-awful and is super contagious (wash your hands!). If your daycare provider sees a speck of goop in your kiddo's eye, I can almost guarantee you're coming to see me before she'll be allowed to go back. This creates some pressure to always treat conjunctivitis. Fortunately, it's often caused by a virus that doesn't require treatment.

ALL ABOUT CONJUNCTIVITIS

- The conjunctiva is the film that covers the pink inside of the eyelids and the white part of the eyeball. This is what gets infected and inflamed.
- It's estimated that about six million people, the majority of whom are children, get conjunctivitis in the United States each year.[69]

- There are three main types: allergic, viral, and bacterial. Allergic conjunctivitis causes very watery and itchy red eyes, often with some swelling of the eyelids as well. It is not contagious and can be improved with allergy eye drops and oral antihistamines. Viral conjunctivitis usually comes along with other viral cold symptoms such as runny nose, sore throat, and cough. Bacterial conjunctivitis can accompany a cold virus or develop completely on its own.

HOW CAN YOU TELL IF IT'S VIRAL OR BACTERIAL?

- Both are likely to make the whites of the eyes red, and they can cause some *mild* swelling of the eyelids as well (it's hard to know if this is from the infection or eye rubbing). Kids often appear comfortable during either type of infection.
- Viral conjunctivitis usually causes thin, almost watery white discharge that is most obvious in the corners of the eyes after waking from sleep. After you wipe it away, it could take hours for the white stuff to come back. Viral infections almost always affect both eyes.
- Bacterial conjunctivitis causes thick, nasty goop buildup that is usually yellow or almost green. When your child wakes up, her eyelids might be matted shut. Bacterial infections often start in just one eye but can quickly spread to the other—kids just can't resist rubbing. After you clean the eye, it keeps churning out goop that needs to be wiped away every hour or so.

WHAT CAN YOU DO TO HELP?

- Keep the infected eye clean with a warm wet washcloth.
- You may have heard the expression "rub some dirt on it"? Well, for infants we say "rub some breast milk on it".

- Even if you're not a fastidiously clean person, this is a time for the entire family to be anal about hand washing. Remember that these germs live on surfaces for a while, so wiping things down with antibacterial spray will help prevent the infection from spreading.

- Bacterial infections need to be treated with antibiotic eye drops (or ointment for infants). Kids three years old and younger should definitely see their doctor because they have a decent chance (about 25 percent) of having an ear infection as well. We assume your child is contagious until she's been treated for twenty-four hours, and most daycares and schools follow this guideline as well. If the infection is borderline, ask your doctor about a prescription to keep on hand in case things worsen.

- Most cases of pink eye are easily treated, but do beware of redness, warmth, and tenderness in the skin around your child's eye. This could be a sign that it has morphed into a skin infection, which is a bigger deal.

WHAT HAPPENED WITH MAISIE?

Mom talks with the pediatric nurse, who recommends coming in because the amount of goop suggests bacterial conjunctivitis. Maisie's doctor finds a pretty impressive left ear infection as well. The doctor treats her with Augmentin, a stronger antibiotic that is the best choice for combo eye-ear infections. Maisie's doing a lot better in two days, but Mom vows not to take her back to Dizzy Castle until she's four.

CROUP

Manny is a chubby-cheeked two-and-a-half-year-old—he looks like he's storing nuts for the long winter. Manny developed a runny nose after waking from his afternoon nap. He ate a bit less for dinner but still seemed pretty happy as he went to bed. Just after midnight, he woke up with a horrible cough unlike anything his parents have heard before. It sounds kind of like a dog or seal barking. He has a fever of 101 and makes a weird sound when he breathes in after a big coughing fit or when he is crying. The sound is like a high-pitched whistle or wheeze, and it goes away when he calms down. His parents give him some ibuprofen for the fever, but what else should they do? They have never heard breathing like that with Manny's colds in the past. Should they take him to the emergency room?

Manny has croup. Croup is common in kids under age six and quite scary when yours gets it for the first time, so it's good to be prepared. Croup is caused by a virus, like other coughs and colds, and as with other viruses, kids get a runny nose and fever. In croup, however, the virus also causes some swelling in the middle of the throat around the vocal cords. That swelling is what makes the cough barky (unmistakable once you've heard it) and causes the wheezy sound with breathing in. The sound, called "stridor," is what can get your child into trouble. Croup is nocturnal—the cough and stridor are always way worse at night. Fortunately, croup is one of the few viral illnesses we can actually do something about! And there are some pretty clear criteria for when your child needs medical attention.

WHAT CAN YOU DO TO HELP?

- Use a humidifier. We're always telling you to use a humidifier for coughs and colds, but for croup it actually makes a big difference. Humidified air soothes the throat and helps the swelling.

- Make a super-humidifier. If your child is having lots of coughing attacks or stridor, go into your smallest bathroom, crank the shower as hot as possible, and make a little steam room.

You can make a mini version of this by draping a towel over both of your heads and leaning over a faucet with the hot water on.

- Bundle him up, and take him outside on the porch to breathe the cool night air. Just like an ice pack on a swollen knee, the cold air will hit his throat and reduce the swelling. If it's a warm summer night, you can use your freezer for a few minutes.

- Give him some ibuprofen. This will help in three ways: First, it will actually reduce the inflammation, unlike acetaminophen. Second, it will bring down the fever. Third, it should make him less fussy, and less crying means less stridor.

WHEN SHOULD YOU WORRY?

It's all about the stridor. The whistling sound happens because he's forcing air through a narrower throat opening. Even when it's just a little bit narrower, you'll hear stridor when your child is pulling big breaths through it (coughing and crying). But if you can hear the whistle with calm, quiet breaths as well, you know his throat is getting pretty tight. If you can't get this to go away with the helpful tricks I mentioned, you need to go to the emergency room. Also, look for the "big eye" sign: If your child is having loud stridor and looking up at you with wide-open scared eyes, you've got to go.

WHEN CAN YOU WAIT IT OUT?

In most cases, the stridor will happen only when he's upset, and you'll be able to control it with steam and cold air. If so, you're safe to stay at home through the night, but you should call your doctor the next morning and be seen. We can give your child a steroid, usually just a single long-lasting dose in the office, that does a terrific job of killing the stridor. Realize that the illness is still caused by a virus, so the steroid won't stop the runny nose and cough from running their course.

WHAT HAPPENED WITH MANNY?

Manny just has stridor when he's upset and coughing, so Mom wraps him up and takes him outside for about five minutes until his breathing is quiet. By the time Dad sets up his humidifier, the ibuprofen is kicking in, and Manny falls asleep. He wakes up again at four in the morning with more stridor, which goes away in the steamy bathroom. Mom brings him in the next morning, and his pediatrician gives him a dose of the long-acting steroid Decadron. The doctor then helps herself to a handful of Manny's cheeks. His stridor is gone the next night, and he continues with a runny nose and barky cough for the next six days.

COUGH

Beckett is a two-year-old whose parents are attending a wedding in Mexico. His dad just got off the phone with Grandma, who's taking care of Beckett, and it sounds like things have not been going well. Beckett spiked a fever of 102 as his parents were boarding the plane, and his symptoms worsened over the next three days. Now he's really congested and his appetite is pretty much gone, but it's the cough that's gotten horrible—it's almost constant and really deep. Grandma says he's breathing faster when he has a fever, but both symptoms improve when she gives him Tylenol. At least he's still playful and drinking okay. What should Dad tell Grandma to do? Give Beckett some cough medicine? Take him to the doctor?

Coughs can sound awful, and everyone knows that lung infections can be quite serious. Most coughs are due to the same viruses that cause cold symptoms, but coughs can also indicate pneumonia, asthma, respiratory syncytial virus (RSV), whooping cough, or other more serious conditions. Some of my worst nights as a parent have been spent lying awake listening to my kids coughing. It's just as frustrating that we can't do a lot to make coughs better most of the time. Fortunately, you can learn to decide if your kid needs help or not.

WHAT'S NORMAL FOR A COUGH?

- It's normal for a cough to sound shallow, deep, throaty, wet, or dry, but how a cough sounds doesn't really tell us much about it. (Aside from a barky cough, which is a pretty good sign of croup—see page 206.) The sound is the first thing that parents bring up (often with a phone recording), but probably the last thing pediatricians ask about.
- It is often worse at night, which is distressing, because it doesn't let your child or you get much sleep. A lot of times this is simply because gunk drains back from his nose and other gunk wants to settle in his lungs.
- It can come in "spurts" or little fits of five or six coughs every now and then. Later we'll distinguish this from "spasms," which are more severe.
- You will often feel rattles or rumbling in your kid's chest or back when he coughs. His lungs are like a big echo chamber, so even when they are crystal clear, you can often feel the rumbling coming from all the goop in the nose and throat.
- Soreness in the throat, stomach muscles, or chest from lots of coughing is very common. Hard coughing is tough on muscles, so some soreness is to be expected.

WHEN SHOULD YOU WORRY?

- When the cough lasts for more than two weeks without any improvement. Coughs are notorious for lingering, but after two weeks there's a higher chance of something going on other than a simple virus, so you should at least check in with your doctor.
- When a cough comes in "spasms." This is more than a spurt. It's a fit of coughing that can go on for a full minute with no relief, to the point where your child turns red in the face and has a hard time catching his breath.

- When your child is working harder to breathe in between coughing episodes. This is the biggie and what I'm most interested in when I see a child with a cough. Is he breathing faster than normal (even when the fever comes down)? Is he using extra muscles to help get air in? There are a few signs of breathing difficulty that most parents can recognize:

  RETRACTIONS. The muscles under and between your child's ribs are getting sucked in every time he breathes so that you can see the ribs more sharply than normal.

  BELLY BREATHING. His tummy is moving in and out with each breath like a pump.

  TRACHEAL TUGGING. That little notch at the bottom of the neck where the collarbones meet gets sucked in with every breath.

  NOSTRIL FLARING. His little nostrils get bigger with each forceful breath.

- When your child is wheezing. This means your child's airways are narrower for some reason. It can be normal with some viruses, especially for infants and toddlers, but it can also be a sign of asthma or certain bacterial infections.
- Symptoms that worsen after a week or after they seemed to be improving. When viruses start to get better, they should keep getting better, so watch out for a fever returning, energy tanking again, or his cough taking another turn for the worse. Those are important signs that need to be checked out.

WHAT CAN YOU DO TO HELP?

- Not much, but you wouldn't know this by going to any store and seeing shelves full of cough medicine. Honey is something safe for toddlers older than twelve months and at least a little helpful according to a 2007 study.[70]

- *Don't* offer your child cough syrup. In contrast to honey, it was *not* found to help in the above study. It feels good to do something for him, and you're going to feel like it probably helps a bit (there's that placebo effect again). But there's no evidence that it works, and cough syrup can be harmful to some kids. If you still decide to use it, be mindful of the age recommendation on the package.
- Use a humidifier. Moist lungs are happy lungs.
- Lots of water! Coughing evaporates fluid, so really push the water.
- Elevate his head. If he's old enough to use a pillow, add an extra one.

WHAT HAPPENED WITH BECKETT?

Beckett has a scary cough, but he's doing okay. Dad calms down when he realizes that his kiddo is breathing fine and staying hydrated. He calls Grandma back and suggests that she get out her old humidifier, give Beckett some honey tonight, and call back tomorrow.

EAR INFECTION

Peyton is a nine-month-old peanut who has been striving for the 5th percentile ever since she was born. She has long sparse wisps of wavy hair that give her the look of a baby mad scientist. She may be small, but she's a firecracker! Peyton has had a cold for the past four days, which she's handled pretty well. She hasn't had a fever; she's just coughing a bit at night and eating less solid food. Her snot has gotten thicker over the past few days. Then last night things blew up—she woke up three times screaming and only finally got back to sleep after some ibuprofen and being held for an hour. She's still clingy the morning after. What's going on? Is it her ears? She doesn't seem to be pulling at them. Should her parents take her in?

Ear infections are a pain. About 50 percent of kids will get at least one by age two, but trying to figure out whether *your* child has one is tough. Until they can say, "Hey, Mom, my left ear hurts," you're just guessing. There are some signs that make an infection more likely, though, and they are worth knowing maybe more than anything else in these case examples, so we'll spend some decent time going over them. One important note: if you suspect an ear infection, try your very best to visit *your* pediatric clinic. Diagnosing and making treatment decisions about them are not straightforward, so a prior familiarity with the child can make a big difference. Urgent care providers who primarily see adults do a lot of things really well, but ear infections are not one of them. It's also important to have the visit records in one place so there is a history of what antibiotics were used and whether ear tubes may be necessary. So if it's 10:00 p.m. and your child wakes up in pain, try to tide her over with ibuprofen and get into your doctor's office the next day.

WHAT ARE THE SIGNS?

- A current or very recent illness. Something has to put the fluid there before it can get infected! Your child's middle ear, right behind the eardrum, is usually filled with air, but colds (or allergies when your child is older) can put fluid in that space instead. There's this little eustachian tube that tries to drain the fluid, but it doesn't always work very well in infants and toddlers. If the fluid sits there long enough, bacteria can turn it into pus. Most ear infections occur at least a few days into a cold when the snot is getting a bit thicker. If your child hasn't had a cold recently, it's *not* an ear infection.

- Fussiness at night is about the best symptom we've got. It's normal to sleep poorly with a cold because of fever or gagging on snot. But an inflamed ear hurts badly when you lay on it. You know your child's pain cry, and if you hear it suddenly a few nights into a cold, you should be thinking ear infection.

- Weird fever patterns. Kids don't get fevers with every virus, but if they do, it usually appears within the first two days of the symptoms starting. Once it goes away for twenty-four hours, it should stay away. So if your child has a cold but gets her first fever on day four of the illness, that can be a sign that fluid somewhere (like the ears) is getting infected with bacteria. I would have the same concern for a fever that goes away after three days but returns two days later.

- Goopy eyes. Infants and toddlers with a bacterial eye infection (pink eye) have a decent chance of getting an ear infection as a result of the same bacteria and should be checked.

- A bunch of nasty stuff draining out of your child's ear. This is the one nobody wants to see. Your child's eardrum can only take so much pressure, so it bursts when there's too much pus behind it. Often you'll see a trail of dried crusty grossness below her ear or on the sheet in the morning. Fortunately the eardrum usually heals well.

WHAT IS *NOT* A SIGN?

- Tugging on the ears. Kids love tugging on and poking their ears. They do it for fun and when they're bored. They do it when they're tired and sometimes to soothe themselves when they're upset. They even do it when they are teething. But on its own, it's *not* a reliable sign of ear infection.

- On and off pain or "plugged" ears in older kids. Kids can get ear infections at any age, but it's a lot less likely after toddlerhood. Pain that comes and goes or plugging usually just points to fluid buildup in the ear.

- Seeing a lot more earwax than normal. Wax doesn't have anything to do with infections because it's outside of the eardrum, and infections are on the inside.

- Getting water in the ear. Sometimes parents are worried because they accidentally splashed dirty water into their child's ear during bath time. But there's no way for that water to get inside the middle ear because the eardrum blocks it.

WHAT CAN YOU DO TO HELP?

- Other than breastfeeding, getting vaccines, and keeping your child away from sick kids, there's nothing you can do to *prevent* ear infections. Decongestants don't help. Putting breast milk, garlic, onion, coconut oil, or essential oils in the ear won't do anything either because there's an eardrum in the way.
- Give your child ibuprofen, which is the most effective over-the-counter medicine for ear pain. Warm compresses over the ear are soothing as well.
- Be patient. Your child *doesn't* always need antibiotics for an ear infection. Severe infections with a lot of pain and fever should probably be treated at any age. Most doctors have a lower threshold for treating more moderate infections under two years of age as well, because these are less likely to clear on their own. But for mild infections, especially in kids over two, we can use a "watchful waiting" strategy. I usually give these parents a prescription with instructions to only start it for worsened pain, increased difficulty sleeping, or new fever. This is a great way to cut down on unnecessary antibiotic use, and it's always okay to ask your doctor if it's an option for your child.

WHAT HAPPENED WITH PEYTON?

Being very fussy at night after a few days of a cold means that Peyton should go in. Her doctor finds a bulging right ear infection, and puts her on seven days of amoxicillin. Her parents get through the next two days with ibuprofen, and by then she perks up, starts sleeping well, and is back to her fiery self.

TIME FOR TUBES?

Many parents worry when their child has had multiple ear infections and wonder whether tubes are needed. Well, it's complicated. Most doctors would agree that kids with six or more infections in a year should get tubes. But usually something else forces our hand. We really only have three antibiotics that are good for treating ear infections, for example, and sometimes they stop working. Fluid in the ears is another problem. Antibiotics should kill the bacteria, but the fluid needs to drain on its own. When it sticks around for weeks or months, your child has a harder time hearing and developing language, which is kind of a big deal. Time of year matters too. If your child has already suffered a bunch of infections and it's only December, I'm a lot more pessimistic than I am if it's April and cold viruses are slowing down.

Ear ventilation tubes (or "PE tubes") are quite common. An otolaryngologist (or ENT—ear, nose, and throat doctor) inserts them into the eardrums with a simple procedure. Nobody wants their child to get a procedure, and there are always risks with general anesthesia, but tubes can be a real game changer for kids struggling with their ears. The tubes often let fluid drain out before it gets infected—and if your kid still gets an infection, you can treat it with ear drops instead of an oral antibiotic.

VOMITING AND DIARRHEA

Dmitri is five months old and smothered with love from his three older sisters. They try to change his outfits about ten times a day and are excited that he finally has enough hair to put bows in. He's thrilled with the attention. Unfortunately, the girls also shared a stomach virus with him. For the past two days he's vomited about three times per day and had about ten watery poops per day. He's been fussy, with a low-grade fever up to 100.8. Dmitri is nursing less than usual and totally refusing to eat the purees he started a few weeks ago. Today Mom is worried because he's only peed twice since yesterday afternoon, and he seems a bit lethargic. She's concerned that Dmitri might be dehydrated. Should she take him to the doctor? To the emergency room?

Being up all night with a vomiting child is one of the toughest experiences you can have as a parent. It usually hits suddenly, and there's not much you can do to stop it, so it's easy to panic. Vomiting and diarrhea are caused by infection and inflammation of your child's stomach and intestines. The fancy term for this is *gastroenteritis*. It's usually caused by a virus but can be caused by bacteria as well. Always remember there's really only one way that vomiting and diarrhea can hurt your kid: *dehydration*. We'll focus on recognizing it, treating it at home, and knowing when you need some help.

WHAT ARE THE SIGNS?

- Vomiting usually starts before diarrhea. It typically lasts for only one or two days, but it can be pretty intense.
- Diarrhea follows shortly after but usually lasts longer, often three to five days. With some viruses (like rotavirus and norovirus), your child can have more than ten episodes of diarrhea per day.
- Kids can develop a fever for up to five days.
- The worst part of the illness can be the cramping abdominal pain that comes and goes. This can be intense and is often relieved by pooping.

WHEN SHOULD YOU WORRY?

- If there is blood in your child's diarrhea. This increases the possibility of a more serious bacterial infection.
- If the vomiting is not improving after two days, or the diarrhea is not improving after four days. (Note: It very well might last longer, but *improving* is the key word.)
- If your child has *severe*, constant pain rather than the on-and-off crampy pain that's expected.
- Your child is peeing a lot less. A bit less than normal is expected during an illness, but if he's down to three or fewer wet diapers (or trips to the potty for older toddlers) per twenty-four hours, that's a sign that his body doesn't have enough fluid.
- Your child cries but doesn't make tears, or his mouth seems dry and "cottony."
- For infants, the "soft spot" on the skull can look more sunken in than normal.
- One of my favorite tests for dehydration is to squeeze the blood out of your child's fingertips and see how long it takes for the red color to return. It should flash back in one or two seconds. If it takes longer, your child's body is low on fluid. His body wants to keep fluid near the big important organs in the middle of the body, so it decreases blood flow to the fingertips.
- Your child is *lethargic*. We talked about how that's a scary word you shouldn't throw around, but dehydration can cause it. Lethargic means that he isn't moving very much and seems weak. He's *too exhausted* to be clingy and is not as interactive with you.

HOMEMADE ORAL REHYDRATION SOLUTION

If you don't have Pedialyte on hand, you can easily make your own version according to the following recipe:

6 flat teaspoons sugar
½ teaspoon table salt
1 liter lukewarm water

Stir all ingredients together in a mason jar or plastic container, and shake or whisk until totally dissolved. Here's a hint—if you need a bit of flavor, you could replace the 6 teaspoons of sugar with about 7 ounces of standard grape or apple juice, with water added to still total one 1 liter of fluid.

WHAT CAN YOU DO TO HELP?

- Give your child probiotics. I would start them at the first sign of diarrhea. There's good evidence that they can reduce the duration of diarrhea by an entire day, which is a big deal.
- Address the cramping. Warm packs on the abdomen and Tylenol work best.
- Consider a prescription for ondansetron (Zofran). This anti-nausea medicine has been used more and more in the past decade. It is *not* necessary for most viruses but can be useful when your child has nausea and vomiting that are not improving.
- Avoid anti-diarrhea medicines (such as Imodium). These basically paralyze the intestines for a while, but you want your child to poop all that virus out.
- Don't restrict his diet too much. The BRAT diet (bananas, rice, applesauce, toast) has been recommended forever to ease a kid's tummy back from an illness, but it's never really

been shown to have any benefit and is too limited. Once he's ready to eat, give him healthy foods that appeal to him (even dairy is okay).

- Don't let it spread! Gastroenteritis tears through households more easily than colds. It is spread by germy hands, and the virus can linger on surfaces for some time. So insist on lots of hand washing, sanitizers, and wipe downs of play areas.

WHAT IF YOUR CHILD IS DEHYDRATED?

Most of the time, we can rehydrate kids orally rather than having to give them IV fluids. If you can get comfortable with doing this at home, you're going to feel more confident during those all-night vomiting sessions and have fewer trips to the doctor. Especially for infants and toddlers, using an "oral rehydration solution" for significant dehydration is crucial. Pedialyte (also available in generic forms) is the classic, but you can also make your own in a pinch (see page 218). Your child loses a lot of salts and electrolytes (like sodium and potassium) in diarrhea and vomit, and oral rehydration solutions replace those. Water, breast milk, and formula are good options for mild stomach viruses when your child is not dehydrated, but they don't replace enough of the salts when vomiting and diarrhea become more severe. Juice and even sports drinks have too much sugar to adequately hydrate your child.

The following rehydration regimen is based on recommendations from the CDC.[71] It is a good place to start, but you need to call your doctor if your child's symptoms are scaring you. In the emergency room, the doctor might calculate the exact amount of fluids your child needs and for how long. At home, just take it hour by hour and see how things go. You can tweak it as needed—the take-home message is *really frequent* and *small* sips.

- Give 5 milliliters of oral rehydration solution by mouth every two minutes for one hour. A syringe is usually the easiest way to give this. That will add up to 5 ounces over an hour. If your child vomits at any point, wait fifteen minutes before resuming rehydration.

- After the first hour, take a fifteen-minute break.
- For the second hour, give 5 to 10 milliliters every two minutes depending on your child's size. Continue this regimen until your child perks up and the signs of dehydration improve.
- If this regimen is interrupted three or more times by vomiting during the first two hours, call your doctor; your child may need IV fluids.

WHAT HAPPENED WITH DMITRI?

Dmitri's mom brings him into the office. His pediatrician diagnoses him with mild dehydration because he's peeing less, has a faster heart rate, and takes about three seconds to get blood back into his fingertips after they're pressed. They start oral rehydration in the office, and Dmitri takes 5 milliliters every two minutes for about an hour without vomiting. He perks up after this and has a decent wet diaper. The doctor lets them go home and tells Mom to do two more hours of oral rehydration and start some probiotics. Dmitri doesn't vomit anymore, and his diarrhea goes away over the next two days. His sisters celebrate by dressing him up like a princess and coloring his toenails with a permanent purple marker.

FEVER

Maricela is twenty months old and an avid climber. She prefers to walk on tables, counters, and couches rather than floors. Perhaps coincidentally, her favorite thing to say is "Gidoff dat!" Maricela is sick. She's had a fever for six days that has spiked as high as 103. Mom can bring it down with Tylenol. She's had some congestion but not much of a cough. Her eyes have been a little red and watery but not goopy. She's drinking okay and still peeing normally. She's very tired and doesn't want to play even when her fever is down. She acts like her legs bother her too. Mom called the clinic three days ago and was told to call back if her fever wasn't gone by today. Now she's really worried and calls first thing in the morning for an appointment.

Fever is a natural response that means your child's body is working to fight an infection. But it's still frightening. In general, your child's breathing and hydration are more important than how high the fever is. But what about when fever is the main symptom? How long is too long? When should we worry? The pattern and duration of the fever can tell us a lot, so let's make it less scary.

As a refresher, a fever is 100.4 degrees Fahrenheit (38 degrees Celsius) or higher. Sorry, 99.5 is not a fever, even if your kid "tends to run at 97." I hear that a lot, but fevers aren't relative. For older kids, armpit, mouth, ear, and temporal artery (forehead scanning) thermometers are all fine—the temporal ones are particularly nice because they're quick and accurate. You'll hear things about adding a degree for certain methods, but don't do that. Sometimes parents tell me that their child was "burning up" but they didn't get a measurement. That's okay, but having the number is nice whenever possible so we can follow trends.

WHAT ARE THE SIGNS?

- It is normal for a fever to start one to two days before or after other symptoms of an illness appear. So if your child is at 101 but doesn't have a runny nose yet, just sit tight and watch her.

- It's also common to have a fever that spikes up past 103. Those high numbers might be scary, but they don't mean that your child has a more severe illness.
- It can climb higher during the evening and nighttime. Viral fevers often do this.
- Fever itself can cause other symptoms too. Your child will breathe a lot faster with a fever. You might feel her heart racing. She can go back and forth between shaking chills and throwing the covers off. With higher fevers your child can be a bit loopy, or "out of it" as well.

WHAT CAN YOU DO TO HELP?

- If your child is uncomfortable, you should treat her. There's a myth out there that a fever helps "cook" the virus and should run its course. That's not really true. In general, kids eat, drink, and play more when their fevers are down. But if she's at 101 and smiling, you can just keep an eye on it.
- You can offer your child acetaminophen (Tylenol) every four hours or ibuprofen (Motrin or Advil) every six. Try to stick with one or the other. However, if the fever comes raging back before the minimum time interval, it's okay to switch to the other medicine. Avoid giving the next dose automatically every four to six hours so you can find out if the fever comes back. We want to get a temperature reading and know what the fever is doing.
- If your kid is at 103 or higher, think about wiping her down with lukewarm wet washcloths either in bed or the bath to help evaporate some of that heat quickly. (Remember that it takes about thirty minutes for the meds to kick in.)

WHEN SHOULD YOU WORRY?

- When a fever lasts longer than five days. Most viral fevers go away within this time.
- When you cannot bring the fever down, despite giving your child fever reducers or a lukewarm bath. If it's only dropping from 103 to 102.5, there's a better chance that bacteria are driving it.
- If the fever has lasted for more than forty-eight hours but no other symptoms have appeared, at least check in with your doctor. It's still probably a virus (such as roseola; see page 235), but we would want to rule out "hidden" causes like urinary tract infections.
- If the fever starts more than forty-eight hours after the other symptoms appear, or if the fever goes away for a full twenty-four hours and then comes back. These can both mean that something somewhere is getting infected. This is often how we discover an ear infection or pneumonia, for example.

WHAT HAPPENED WITH MARICELA?

Maricela's pediatrician is worried about her because her fever has lasted for six days without many other symptoms, and she looks crummy. He decides to get some bloodwork to look for signs of bacterial infection or inflammation. Fortunately, the bloodwork is reassuring, and it appears to just be an especially nasty virus. The doctor calls Maricela's mom to check in the next day and learns that her fever has finally broken. He is even more relieved to hear Mom yell, "Maricela! Get off that!"

FEBRILE SEIZURE

These are uncommon—only about 2 to 5 percent of kids under six years old will ever experience one. However, they are scary, so I want you to be aware of them. They can happen with *high* fevers, usually above 103, and especially when the fever spikes quickly. Here's a scenario: you're already really concerned about your sick kid, and then she has a true seizure that often involves her entire body shaking. You can't stop the shaking, which can last for a few minutes. She doesn't respond to you during this time, and even after the shaking stops, she'll be groggy for a while. Watching this unfold is absolutely terrifying, but believe it or not, it usually isn't dangerous to your child. Most parents end up calling 911, but if the seizure lasts fewer than five minutes, it's okay to wait it out and then check in with your doctor. Kids who have one febrile seizure have a 30 percent chance of experiencing another one at some point, and they have a *very slightly* increased risk of epilepsy when they are older (about 2 percent versus 1 percent for the rest of the population).

CONSTIPATION

Kingston is a big four-year-old boy whose main hobby is imitating superheroes. He's really kind of quiet until he puts a cape on. . . . Then he swoops around the house, flies through the supermarket, and jumps off tables at the library—all while doing impressive sound effects. Through several years of experimentation, he has found the ideal superhero fuel to be a delicate blend of crackers, bread, cheese, and chicken nuggets. For the past two weeks he's been complaining of pain below his belly button at random times. It makes him bend over sometimes and lasts for ten to fifteen minutes. He hasn't had any fever, vomiting, or diarrhea. He poops every day and it never seems to hurt him, but he's finally started wiping himself over the past few months (thank God), so his dad doesn't really know how it looks. Kingston's appetite is normal, and he's otherwise been really healthy. What's going on? Is it a food allergy? A weird stomach bug? Does he just want attention? He's usually not a complainer. Is it time to get it checked out?

It's hard to know what to do with tummy pain sometimes. Kids have sensitive stomachs, and there is a long list of things that can upset them. Also, it's difficult for little kids to express when they feel shy, nervous, or sad, but they know how to say their tummy hurts from a young age. Sometimes that's their way of saying they just don't feel right. Then they very much notice that they get some love and attention when they tell you it hurts, which makes it even harder to know when you should actually be concerned. One fact will always be true, however—when it comes to tummy pain in kids under five, constipation is the undisputed champion. It's hard to exaggerate how common it is or how many problems it can cause. It can be tough to discover, though, since many affected kids still poop every day and older toddlers are wiping and flushing on their own. Let's figure it out.

WHAT ARE THE SIGNS?

- Your child has brought up tummy pain without prompting every day for a week. Constipation builds up over time and causes daily symptoms, so take this seriously.

- Discomfort comes while your child is playing or doing something really fun. To me, this is always the best way to see if something is bothering him or if he's just seeking attention. Real problems can happen at *any* time, not just when your child is bored.
- The pain is crampy, which makes your child want to bend over with his arm across his lower abdomen. This type of pain usually comes in ten- to fifteen-minute bursts (when the intestines are squeezing) and then might go away for an hour or more (when the intestines are relaxing).
- The pain seems worse after your child eats. When you eat, your intestines wake up and squeeze to make room for the new food coming through. When they squeeze on hard poop, it hurts.
- It starts to affect your child's appetite or behavior. If left untreated, constipation can decrease appetite, cause nausea, and even worsen behavior. It can even affect your child's peeing too, causing it to be more frequent and painful and making infections more likely.
- Your child is pooping less often than he used to, taking longer to poop, or trying to poop but failing sometimes. Hard poop, which tends to look pebbly, is also a warning sign.
- There are small thin streaks of blood on the stool. This is often caused by little cracks in the anal area when your child passes a really big hard stool. Larger amounts or persistent blood always need to be investigated further.

WHAT CAN YOU DO TO HELP?

- Give your child Miralax. For most pediatricians, constipation treatment starts with this super-safe over-the-counter medicine (generic name: polyethylene glycol). It's a powder that has no taste, and it works by pulling water into your child's intestine to soften the poop. Dosage is approximate: It comes with a measuring cap, and a full cap per day is a regular adult dose.

OTHER CAUSES OF STOMACH PAIN

ANXIETY. If you notice that your child has pain only on preschool days or when he's going to soccer class, for example, it's probably anxiety. This real pain can come with some loose poops as well, and it's probably the second most common cause after constipation. Reassurance that the pain will improve as he gets more comfortable in new situations is usually all you need to offer.

LACTOSE INTOLERANCE. If your child's pain tends to come after he consumes dairy and includes gassiness and loose stools, he may be dealing with some lactose intolerance. This tends to appear around ages four to five. If you're suspicious, talk to your doctor or try removing dairy from your child's diet for ten days (you can use Lactaid or other alternative milks during this time as needed). Milk and ice cream are the toughest to tolerate, but most kids do fine with moderate amounts of cheese or yogurt.

ACID REFLUX. If your child complains of burning in his chest, pain that's worse when lying down, or a yucky taste in his mouth, this can indicate that stomach acid is washing up and down the esophagus. Reflux is pretty common for babies and even teenagers, but not so much for toddlers. Talk to your doctor if you're concerned.

"FUNCTIONAL ABDOMINAL PAIN." What if you've explored all of the main offenders and nothing seems to fit? Then we're left with this diagnosis, which is basically the pediatric equivalent of irritable bowel syndrome. These means that your kid has pain without any obvious cause and maybe even normal labs or studies, but he is still thriving and gaining great weight. A little reassuring and a little frustrating.

If your child is below age two, talk to your doctor about the appropriate amount. If your child is over two, it's reasonable to start with a half cap per day and adjust as needed to get one or two soft stools per day. I always recommend about two weeks of consistent treatment to get your child back on track—if the constipation returns after you stop it, it's safe to be on it for months at a time.

- Make changes to your child's diet. This is also important, but probably more of a long-term project. Kids who eat lots of starchy foods, processed foods, dairy, and bananas tend to get constipated. Increasing water and foods with fiber such as veggies and fruits helps.
- Consider a full cleanout. If your child is severely constipated, your doctor might recommend a "cleanout" using a few different medicines and maybe even enemas over a weekend to get things going.

Your child's tummy ache is almost never due to food allergies! This is a common concern for parents, but food allergies are usually going to show up with more intense symptoms that get worse over time, like hives or severe abdominal pain with vomiting within thirty minutes of eating a food.

Finally, there is a long list of scary things that can cause stomach pain, but a very small chance that your child has any of them. Obviously, call your doctor if your kid has persistent or large amounts of blood in the stool, or if his pain is severe. For me, energy level is a huge sign. Kids should have tons of energy. If your kid is consistently complaining of pain and seems to be more tired than usual, check in with your doctor.

WHAT HAPPENED WITH KINGSTON?

Even though Kingston poops every day, his starch- and dairy-heavy diet, along with his crampy on-and-off pain, make constipation the likely diagnosis. Dad puts him on one-half cap of Miralax per day, and after four days his pain goes away. Kingston is so thrilled that he puts three capes on at once and flies off the dining room table. Dad continues giving him Miralax for two weeks and replaces some of the superhero's carb-heavy snacks with real superfoods: water, fruits, and vegetables.

VAGINITIS OR URINARY TRACT INFECTION?

Sophia is a three-year-old with frizzy red hair and a pony obsession. She has about twenty ponies and actually cleaned her room once to make space for the real one she's expecting for her fourth birthday. Her parents send her and her team to Grandma's house on a Friday to stay over. Sophia returns the next morning smelling like jelly donuts and complains that it hurts when she pees. She doesn't have a fever and she's still eating fine, but she runs to the bathroom every twenty minutes. She cries on the potty and only a few drops come out. She's scratching her genitals a lot but doesn't have a fever or otherwise seem sick. Mom's nervous—is this a UTI? It's Saturday afternoon and the doctor's office is closed. What should she do?

This is a tough one. Urinary infections are fairly common between ages two and six, when girls are working on wiping and good hygiene. It's important to catch those quickly before they become a more serious kidney infection and a trip to the doctor is necessary. But vaginitis (a.k.a. vulvovaginitis) is even more common at this age. Vaginitis is irritation in the vaginal and urethral area caused by a wide variety of things—poor hygiene, soaps, shampoos, sweat, friction. Kids then get caught in a cycle where scratching, wiping, soap, and urine keep the irritation going. And even though it's more common in girls, boys can get similar irritation near their urethra. Here are some hints on distinguishing between the two conditions and breaking the cycle of vaginitis.

WHAT ARE THE SIGNS OF VAGINITIS?

- An urgency to pee, which means that your child feels like she has to suddenly go really badly, but when she gets to the toilet only a few drops come out. This can happen often, like several times per hour.

- Pain or burning when she's actually peeing due to the salty urine coming into contact with the irritated tissue around the urethra.

- Redness of the tissue around the urethra. (UTIs are completely internal—they don't make the outside of the body red.)
- Your child might scratch her genitals a lot or readjust her underwear.

WHEN SHOULD YOU WORRY ABOUT A UTI?

- If your child has a fever, especially if she doesn't have any cold symptoms to blame it on.
- If your child is tired, has a decreased appetite, is vomiting, or otherwise looks sick.
- If she complains about pain in her stomach or back, even when she isn't peeing.
- If there's a really bad smell to her urine that you don't recognize.
- If your child experiences severe pain when she pees, sometimes to the point that she avoids going.

WHAT CAN YOU DO TO HELP?

- It all starts with sitz baths. This means having your child sit in a clean bathtub with water and nothing else, not even baby soap or shampoo. Try to do this twice a day for two or three days.
- Put petroleum jelly on anything that looks red to protect it from the salty urine, sweat, and friction that can keep the problem going.
- For wiping, either wet the toilet paper and dab, or rinse out some unscented baby wipes and keep them in a ziplock bag. You can also clean your child off after she pees by flushing her genitals with a water bottle filled with warm water. The whole point is to avoid friction.
- Good hydration: the less salty the urine, the less it will burn.

WHAT HAPPENED WITH SOPHIA?

On further questioning, Mom finds out that Grandma treated Sophia to a bubble bath using Mr. Bubble soap left over from Mom's childhood. Bubble bath solutions are notorious for causing vaginitis, especially when they are thirty years old. Since Sophia has no fever and does not seem sick, a UTI is unlikely. Mom focuses on sitz baths and some of the other techniques to break the cycle of irritation. After two days, the pony princess is good as new.

RASH

Jonah is a three-and-a-half-year-old golf fanatic. His parents have never played a round in their lives, but Jonah got a few plastic clubs for his birthday and found that he rather liked whacking things with them. Now he can drive the ball fifty yards, enjoys wearing pastels, and forces his parents to record major PGA Tour events. He's been spending a lot of time outside this summer working on his stroke. Over the past week, his parents have noticed a bumpy red rash on his lower arms, legs, and neck. The rash is really itchy, but he's otherwise completely healthy. No one else in the family has a rash, and Jonah hasn't been tromping around in the woods. Mom tries some lotion, but it doesn't seem to help much. Her friend says it's probably a food allergy (has she tried cutting out gluten?), but Mom decides to set up an appointment with her pediatrician.

Skin is weird. It's amazing at protecting us and healing quickly when it's damaged, but sometimes it goes haywire. Rashes are extremely common and often really tough to figure out. And I think parents universally get freaked out by rashes because they know that a few of them can indicate scary things. Fortunately, most rashes are mild and go away on their own. And remember that *how your child is doing* is always more important than how peculiar the rash looks. There's a lot to cover here, so let's get started.

WHAT ARE SOME COMMON RASHES?

- HEAT RASH. You'll see little red bumps, maybe a bit raised, that tend to appear on your child's "trunk" (chest, stomach, and back). This is caused by his little sweat glands getting plugged up and slightly irritated. You might notice it when he's been in his car seat for a while on a warm day. Heat rash never bothers him and usually goes away within a day.

- VIRAL RASH. These rashes are common and usually come along with a fever early in the course of a virus (roseola being an exception; see page 235). They often consist of flat red dots that are mostly on the trunk. Most are not itchy and tend to resolve after three days. If your child is doing well and has obvious viral symptoms, you are probably fine watching this at home.

- CONTACT DERMATITIS. This is irritation from or sensitivity to something that comes into physical contact with your child's skin. The classic example is poison oak or ivy. Other common causes are laundry detergents, fabric softeners, sunblocks, soaps, shampoos, and lotions. Often it's the perfumes or dyes in these products that cause the irritation. This rash can make the skin look bubbly and weepy when severe or just cause some slightly raised red bumps. Also, look for a pattern. If it's from sunblock, for example, it might spare the areas that a shirt and shorts cover. You might see rash on the scalp, neck, and shoulders if shampoo is the culprit.

- ECZEMA. See page 237 for more about this common inflammatory skin condition.

- HIVES. See page 200 for more about this allergic reaction.

- INSECT BITES: Plenty of critters cause rashes. Everyone knows what mosquito bites look like, but a lot of other bites just cause little nondescript red bumps. What insect bites have in common is that they are *itchier* than most other rashes. Figure out whether your child is developing new bumps day after day. If so, that might implicate critters living in your house (fleas, bed bugs, body lice, scabies, etc.). I'll bet it makes you itchy just thinking about it, but it has nothing to do with how clean your home is, and your pediatrician can help you figure it out.

- "RINGWORM." This is a confusing name because it's also the name of a parasite that infects dogs, but the skin ringworm that your child can get is really a fungus called *tinea corporis*. He can get it from other kids and surfaces such as playmats. It usually starts as a faint oval ring. As it progresses, it gets kind of scaly (and less red) in the middle and often develops a slightly raised red ring around the border. It's usually slightly itchy. This fungus isn't dangerous, but it's annoying and takes a while to treat. The most important thing is to stay on top of it before it spreads.

- IMPETIGO. This sounds like a tropical disease, but it's actually a common superficial infection caused by strep and staph bacteria. It likes the skin around kids' mouths and noses, especially if they already have some skin breakdown or rash. It can look like a goopy yellow crust ("honey-colored" is what we're taught) or come in tiny little bubbles that are clustered together. Around the nostrils it can look like crusty boogers. It's not usually dangerous, but it can spread, so see the doctor if you think your child has it.

- CELLULITIS/ABSCESS. These deeper bacterial infections are bad news, and they have become more common as nasty, drug-resistant bugs such as MRSA have become the norm in many places. Cellulitis can start at a scrape or insect bite and then spread through a deeper layer of skin. An abscess is a pocket of infection that can fill with pus and spread *deep* into the skin. It usually has a bump you can feel, sometimes with a whitehead. Three big keys to these infections should prompt you to get your kid in to see the doctor: the skin is *red*, *warm*, and *tender*. Your child may even have a fever. These infections spread shockingly fast and most need oral antibiotics.

WHAT CAN YOU DO TO HELP?

- KEEP THE SKIN MOIST. Remember that your child's skin is a better barrier when it is hydrated. So even if he doesn't need lotion normally, rashy skin usually likes lotion. It is always most effective right after a bath before the skin has a chance to dry.
- CONTROL THE ITCHING. Scratching a rash can feel *so* good. Admit it—you can't help yourself! Neither can your kid. But scratching just causes a cycle of more itching, redness, and scratching. It can also spread certain types of rashes and damage your child's skin, making him vulnerable to infection. For small areas, hydrocortisone cream (the weak one available over the counter should do) works better than Benadryl (diphenhydramine) cream. A cold washcloth is great, and band-aids can keep the rash out of sight and out of mind. When the itchiness is winning, you may have to bring in the big guns—oral Benadryl every four to six hours.
- WATCH THE HEAT. When your child gets hot, the tiny little blood vessels in his skin will open up to cool him off. But they'll also release a bunch of the chemicals that make his rash redder and itchier. So keep baths lukewarm.
- GET A JUMPSTART ON MILD INFECTIONS. If you are suspicious of ringworm, start using clotrimazole cream (Lotrimin), which is available over the counter. If the skin is breaking down from scratching, try some antibiotic ointment (it may require a prescription ointment if it starts to look worse).

WHEN SHOULD YOU WORRY?

- When a rash is hot, red, and painful, or when it comes with a fever but no other viral symptoms. These can be signs of infection.

- When the rash doesn't "blanch." Most rashes blanch, which means you can press the redness out of them with a finger and it returns quickly after you lift your finger. If you're having a hard time telling, take a clear glass with a flat bottom and press it against the rash. The skin should appear white while you're doing this.
- When it happens while your child is taking a medication. Sometimes this is a coincidence, but we need to make sure it's not an allergy.

VIRAL RASHES TO RECOGNIZE!

There are a few viruses that cause rash that are worth mentioning. They all have specific patterns that you can easily distinguish. And they all look a lot worse than they are. You can save yourself a lot of grief, panic, and doctor visits if you get familiar with them.

ROSEOLA. If I were British, I'd say roseola was a bugger. It's quite common in younger kids, especially under age two, and it hits suddenly with a high fever that often reaches 103 or 104. When his fever's down, your child looks pretty good with no other major symptoms—maybe a slightly runny nose or loose poops. But this makes everyone nervous, because we like to have a reason for fevers. The fever usually lasts for about three days. The day after it goes away your child often gets a red rash most visible on his chest, stomach, and back. That pattern is the key, because most viral rashes come during (not after) the fever. But *you're* going to be relieved when you see that rash and say, "Oh, it was just roseola." It will be gone after a few days, and then your kid's back in business.

Continued on next page . . .

Continued from previous page . . .

FIFTH DISEASE. When you read about this illness, a picture of some cute kid with rosy cheeks and a big smile on her face always accompanies it. It starts with a "slapped-cheek rash" that can be a bit warm to the touch. Kids usually feel pretty good otherwise, with maybe some mild cold symptoms, tiredness, or low-grade fever. After a few days, many kids also get a lacy pink rash on their body, most notably the arms. The rash fades after about a week. One warning about this mild illness, though—the parvovirus that causes it is *not* good for pregnant women.

HAND, FOOT, AND MOUTH DISEASE. Oh, the humanity! This sounds like some kind of mad cow disease or leprosy or something. It is the scourge of daycares and preschools, and it often peaks during the summer or fall. It frequently starts with a fever and your kid feeling kind of crummy (unlike roseola or fifth disease). Shortly after the fever, most kids get red spots or bumps on their hands and feet, as well as around their mouths and groin areas. These bumps can turn into purplish, nasty-looking blisters as well. Kids get similar sores in their throats that look like canker sores. These are what really make them miserable. Some kids can have enough throat sores to make drinking tough, so good hydration is the most important thing you can do to help. The illness resolves on its own after about a week, but don't be surprised when your child's fingers or nails start peeling a few weeks later.

- If you are having a hard time controlling the itching and/or scratching.
- If the rash is not improving after about three days.

WHAT HAPPENED WITH JONAH?

Jonah's pediatrician notices that the rash really seems to spare his trunk and his upper arms and legs. He asks Mom about sunblock, and Mom recalls that she started using a new one that smells like coconuts a few weeks ago. The pediatrician diagnoses him with contact dermatitis and recommends using a hypoallergenic product instead. He recommends Benadryl as needed for the itching and prescribes a mild steroid cream as well. The rash is gone four days later, and Mom shifts her attention to the crack in the TV left by a textbook indoor swing.

ECZEMA

Delia is an eight-month-old girl with vibrant green eyes. For some reason, she loves people with lots of hair—the poofier the better. Unfortunately, her dad is quite bald. Sometimes he'll pull out an old wig he wore to a disco party once to make her giggle. Delia has always had sensitive skin. She's usually rashy in the "drool zone," and if you pick her up, you can see the finger marks for a while. But over the past three weeks her skin has looked a lot worse. She has developed red rough patches over her cheeks, stomach, outer legs, and wrists. The rash seems to bother her—she'll rub at her cheeks and sometimes Dad sees new scratches on her wrists when she wakes up in the morning. Dad has been racking his brain trying to figure out the cause. They did start yogurt around that time, but all the soaps, shampoos, and detergents haven't changed. He's been putting some lavender lotion on her skin every morning, but it doesn't seem to be helping much. What's going on? Does she need medicine? He feels like if he can make her rash go away he might finally win her over, hair or not . . .

At least 10 percent of kids in the United States are diagnosed with eczema, and in my experience it's even more common in babies. It can be very itchy, and babies are surprisingly good at scratching with their chubby little fingers. You can think of eczema as hyper-reactive skin. When something like dryness or sweat irritates the skin of someone with eczema, the skin goes overboard and sends all kinds of chemicals to fight the irritation. But the chemicals do more harm than good and just make the skin red and itchy. Unlike a lot of other rashes, you can't eliminate eczema—you just control it. The key is breaking that cycle of itching and scratching.

WHAT ARE THE SIGNS?

- Location, location, location. As kids get older, eczema really likes creases, especially the elbows, knees, and wrists. It's a bit different in babies, though. They tend to get it on their faces, over the outsides of their arms and legs, and on their trunk. A real hint is if it involves the creases behind the ears.
- Eczema often comes in somewhat oval-shaped patches but can consist of more widespread bumps. More than that, you can *feel* it. It's always rough or bumpy.
- It's *itchy*!
- It doesn't go away very quickly with lotion. Most rashes caused by something irritating, like those in the "drool zone" around the mouth and upper chest, get better after just one or two days of petroleum jelly or healing ointment. Eczema tends to be self-sustaining once it flares.

WHAT CAN YOU DO TO HELP?

Lots. Remember, we control eczema rather than cure it. We'll divide treatment into maintenance that you continue every day even when your child's skin looks great, and how to handle flare-ups. I consider a flare-up to be redness or itching (or both) that starts even when you're doing the maintenance regimen. That implies a bad cycle is starting, and you will want to stop it as quickly as possible.

For daily maintenance:

- "Soak and seal." When your child takes a bath and then just dries to the air, her skin ends up *drier*. So after you pat her dry, you want to lock in that moisture with lotion.

- Use lotion *every single day*. You want something thick that doesn't smell like anything. We've already talked about good daytime options like Eucerin or Cetaphil that rub all the way into the skin. During especially dry times, you can always ramp up to twice a day or use an even thicker ointment like Vaseline or Aquaphor.

- Avoid irritants. Eczema skin is usually happier with "free and clear" detergents and sunblock that doesn't smell tropical. After swimming, make sure to rinse off the chlorine, and don't use bubble bath. Just common sense stuff.

For any flare-ups:

- Topical steroids are *absolutely essential* for kids with anything beyond mild eczema. You always want the weakest one that works well. Sometimes the super-weak hydrocortisone 1% that you can buy over the counter is enough for babies, but most kids need something stronger that your doctor can prescribe. People are afraid of steroids, so most start them too late and stop them too early. During a flare-up, always apply it twice per day right away and do an extra day after the skin looks good again. This will let the skin heal and give you a longer time until the next flare-up. If three days of steroid ointment doesn't start to improve the rash, it's time to see your doctor for something stronger.

- Control the itching. It feels great, and it's tough to resist. During a flare-up, try to cover the affected skin with breathable clothes (or a band-aid) and keep fingernails short. Make baths lukewarm. Since a lot of itching happens at night when kids are half-asleep, it's okay to give a bedtime dose of Benadryl for a few nights when things are bad.

WHEN SHOULD YOU WORRY?

- Beware of infection. When skin is red and broken down, bacteria can get in more easily. You need to see your doctor for yellow-orange crusting or lack of improvement with your normal regimen.
- Know that other conditions tend to "travel" with eczema. Your child will be a bit more likely to have allergies (food or environmental) or asthma at some point. These are similar "overreactions" to things that irritate your body.
- Try to avoid elimination diets before talking with your pediatrician. Most kids with mild or moderate eczema are not triggered by foods, so I would recommend against taking dairy, soy, eggs, gluten, or other foods out of her diet (or yours, if breastfeeding) unless you talk with your doctor. It will just drive you crazy.

WHAT HAPPENED WITH DELIA?

Dad takes her in to the pediatrician, who diagnoses Delia with eczema and prescribes a 2.5% hydrocortisone ointment to use for flare-ups. He tells Dad to slather her with Eucerin rather than the lavender lotion following every bath. After three days of this regimen, her skin looks terrific. Delia grabs her dad's bald head with both chubby hands and plants a kiss on him—he's in!

DIAPER RASH

Yumiko is three months old and has just emerged from a haze of colic. Turns out she's actually a pretty sweet girl. Mom is out of town, so Dad's all over it. He's thawing breast milk like a pro, taking her out for walks in the baby carrier, bringing her to his favorite coffee shop—and he's posting photos to his Facebook page to prove it. One day in he takes Yumiko to the zoo and they have a total blast—he makes all the animal sounds, she smiles and coos, it's lots of fun. When they get back to the car, Dad realizes that she has been sitting in a soaked diaper for half the day, which has caused her mild diaper rash to explode. The rash is bright, beefy red, and goes all the way down into her creases. There are some little red dots along the edges of the rash as well. Uh oh. He wants to fix this before Mom returns in two days. Since it's Sunday, he takes a picture and wisely sends it to his pediatrician cousin (rather than Facebook) to get some help.

Diaper rashes are a pain, and most kids in diapers get them from time to time. There are lots of different types and even more treatments you can buy for them. I think parents tend to feel guilty, too, for not changing their kids quickly enough. But even with the best care, sometimes they just happen. Here I identify some of the heavy hitters.

WHAT ARE SOME COMMON DIAPER RASHES, AND HOW SHOULD YOU TREAT THEM?

- "Normal" diaper rash is caused by pee, poop, and sweat, and it probably makes up 90 percent of diaper rashes. Bodily fluids are irritating, and it doesn't take much time for them to make the skin red. These rashes are especially likely to appear with diarrhea and when older infants and toddlers eat acidic foods. The skin usually looks pink or red, and the creases at the top of your child's legs are usually *spared*. Sometimes the skin can actually be broken down and look kind of raw (kind of like the base of a blister that's popped).
    - To treat this type of rash, you want to start applying a diaper rash cream at the first sign of redness. It's great to have one at home with 40 percent zinc oxide (these are white and pasty: Desitin, Boudreaux's Butt Paste, or Balmex). Zinc oxide is a good barrier and hard to rub off. When things get a bit more raw, I really prefer plain petroleum jelly with every diaper change. When the rash seems painful, try some hydrocortisone cream under the diaper cream twice a day. If your baby is eating solids, take it easy on the acidic foods for a few days (tomato, citrus, melon, etc.). Finally, a little time out of the diaper helps a lot. Yes, I realize this is playing with fire.

- A yeast diaper rash is *red* (like fire-engine red) and really likes the genital area. Yeast is everywhere, and it just loves to grow in places that are dark, warm, and moist, like diapers. It loves moving in on top of "normal" diaper rashes, when the skin barrier isn't working so well. It looks like a big red patch with a well-defined border, and there are often little red dots just off of that border. Finally, it usually *loves* a baby's creases, since they are even darker, wetter, and warmer.
    - To treat a yeast rash, apply over-the-counter clotrimazole 1% cream (Lotrimin), which usually takes care of it. Yeast isn't dangerous, just annoying. Some time out of the diaper is especially important. Yeast is so common that I recommend parents try some clotrimazole for any diaper rash that doesn't seem to be improving after three days with the use of regular barrier creams.
- An allergic diaper rash is less common and caused by sensitivity to diapers, creams, wipes, or detergents used to wash cloth diapers. You will see slightly red patches or dots. This is usually more widespread than other diaper rashes. For example, you're more likely to see rash in the area of the diaper band or over little butt cheeks (areas that pee and poop have a harder time getting to). Another hint is that they tend to appear randomly when there has not been any diarrhea or prolonged time in wet diapers. Always ask yourself if you've changed any diaper products recently.
    - Treatment for an allergic rash takes a little bit of detective work. Try switching diapers for a week first if the rash is up by the waistband or in the shape of a diaper. Otherwise, try switching diaper creams or rinsing out the wipes before you use them, even if they are "sensitive" or "all natural." The rash itself should respond well to hydrocortisone.

- Finally, there is bacterial diaper rash, which is less common but a little bit scarier. Like yeast, bacteria are everywhere, and irritated skin is an invitation for them to move in. Infected hair follicles are the most common one for kids in diapers. These are raised red bumps that can be as big as a pencil eraser, sometimes with little whiteheads on them. Superficial infections can also cause crusting, peeling, oozing, or blistering of the skin.
    - To treat this type of rash, you should see your pediatrician, who might suggest antibiotics in ointment or liquid form. If you can't get in for a day, it's always fine to try some over-the-counter antibiotic ointment.

WHAT HAPPENED WITH YUMIKO?

Fortunately, Dad's pediatrician cousin recognizes that Yumiko has a yeast diaper rash and tells him to start using some clotrimazole. He pays extra special care to changing her and watches the rash nearly disappear within two days. When Mom gets home, Yumiko is babbling in delight, and Dad basks in his wife's admiration of a job well done.

STREP THROAT

Matty is a brainy four-year-old who weighs thirty-two pounds soaking wet. He can read pretty well already and specializes in ocean predators. Two days ago he woke up complaining of a sore throat. That evening he developed a fever that peaked at 102. Since yesterday he has been feeling pretty crummy and complaining that his tummy and head hurt. He's drinking okay but not eating much. He doesn't seem very congested and isn't coughing. He's kind of just hanging out on the couch grilling his mom with trivia from his shark encyclopedia. Did you know that the basking shark is the second-biggest fish? His mom is worried that he might have strep throat but she can't get a good look in there. Should she bring him in?

Strep throat is a classic and common illness. Bacteria infect the tissue in the back of the throat, and if you've ever had it, you know it's miserable. Most people think that we treat it to make symptoms go away more quickly, but that's not really true. Giving antibiotics probably knocks a day off the illness, but we mainly treat strep to prevent rheumatic fever. The toxins made by the strep bacteria can cause this illness weeks later, and it can lead to inflamed joints and eventually heart problems. This used to be a common complication and is now quite rare (yay, antibiotics!).

WHAT ARE THE SIGNS?

- A bad sore throat without impressive cold symptoms is the biggest sign and something you should remember. Sore throats are a part of most regular colds. They usually are an early symptom and then fade as the runny nose and cough get worse. But with strep, those cold symptoms just don't come.
- Kids almost always have fever with strep, usually in the 101 to 102 range.
- Tummy pain and headaches. In my experience, young kids with strep complain of this a lot, but without the vomiting and diarrhea.
- Your child looks *saggy*. You've seen how he just powers right through most colds when you keep his fever down. Kids are noticeably tired with strep.
- Your child is at least three years old. Strep is rare before age three, so you usually don't have to worry about testing for it unless a family member has it.
- Lots of white and red spots in the throat. It's hard to look in a kid's throat, so you don't need to worry too much about trying to see back there. *But* bright red spots or what looks like pus in the back of the throat is more common in strep than in viral sore throats.

- A classic strep rash. This is typically not present, but it's pretty unmistakable when it appears—it's a very fine red rash that feels kind of like sandpaper when you rub it. It's usually most obvious on the chest, stomach, and back.

WHAT CAN YOU DO TO HELP?

- Get a prescription for antibiotics. Strep always needs to be treated, and fortunately, it's easy to kill with good old amoxicillin. But don't rush in the first day your child has a sore throat. Remember that cold symptoms can appear a day or two after the sore throat, so waiting can avoid an unnecessary trip. Also, the quick little throat swab that your doctor will do to test for strep is a bit more accurate if you've waited at least twenty-four hours. To prevent the bad stuff that can come after strep, you have at least a week to get treatment.
- Try to control the symptoms. Because there's inflammation in the throat from strep, ibuprofen is a better choice than Tylenol for controlling pain and fever. A humidifier is important to keep the throat moist at night, and lozenges or Chloraseptic spray can soothe as well. As always, hydrate your child like crazy, and don't worry about the eating for a few days.
- Quarantine your child. Strep is very contagious through saliva, and kids are good at slinging it around. He will be contagious until he's been on the antibiotics for at least twenty-four hours, so keep him under wraps.

WHAT HAPPENED WITH MATTY?

Matty's doctor recommends coming in since he has a bad sore throat and fever but no cold symptoms. His throat swab is positive for strep and he gets ten days of "the pink stuff." The doctor says he should be feeling better in about two to three days and recommends laying low in the meantime. On the way out, Matty casually suggests to his doctor that the bull shark might even be more dangerous than the great white due to its ability to hunt in both salt- and freshwater.

Closing Thoughts

It's an incredible thing, being a parent. How can it be so hard and frustrating and exhausting and amazing and loving and fulfilling all at once? Again and again I'm inspired by how anxious new parents become calm, confident parents. You prepare with the best information you can find, surround yourself with people you trust, and make thoughtful decisions. Hopefully this book has helped you to do that. Then you just fall hopelessly in love with your kid every day. Enjoy the next four years—to say they'll fly by is an understatement. In the probable event that you kept nodding off while you read this book (sleep deprivation!), or if you were more of a "CliffsNotes" kind of student back in the day, here's a cheat sheet of the most important aspects of the book:

TOP TEN KEYS TO PARENTING SUCCESS

1. Talk to your baby.
2. Be firm but loving.
3. Worry about *what* your child eats, not *how much*.
4. Sleep train your baby.
5. Watch out for sugar.
6. Put your smartphone down.
7. Turn the TV off.
8. Develop a healthy cynicism about stuff marketed to your kid.
9. Set up a good time-out system for your toddler.
10. Relax—you're doing a great job!

Acknowledgments

I didn't really set out to write a book. My goal was to come up with something for my patients' families to take home after visits since we never have enough time. So I want to thank all the parents and kids I see every day. It's been wonderful getting to know you and watching your kids grow up. This book is for you.

I'd also like to thank my agent, Anne Devlin, for taking a chance on me and working hard to make this book a reality. I'd like to thank the entire team at Sasquatch Books for their support and guidance, especially Susan Roxborough, Rachelle Longé McGhee, Em Gale, and Shari Miranda.

I'd also like to thank Charlie Rapp, Clo Johnson-Beale, Paul Goodwin, Mary Choi, Dana Ben-Artzi, Jean Nava, Dick Cohen, Craig Rubin, and Deborah Rubin for taking the time to read chapters and give me feedback. They are all pediatricians and parents who I respect, and their input was invaluable.

Thanks to Daniel Wilson and Tracy Cutchlow, real live authors who gave me timely advice and motivation. Special thanks to my fellow doctors and the staff at Evergreen Pediatrics, for putting up with me and making work fun while keeping kids first always.

Most of all I'd like to thank my wife, Camille Yu, also a pediatrician and the only one our friends call for advice. Without her support, no-holds-barred editing, and willingness to take the kids while I snuck off to write, this book never would have happened. And finally to Augie and Elsie, who have taught me more about being a parent than anyone. I love you always.

Notes

THE FINAL PREPARATIONS

1. "Cost of Raising a Child Calculator," Center for Nutrition Policy and Promotion, United States Department of Agriculture, accessed January 11, 2018, https://www.cnpp.usda.gov/calculatorintro.

IT'S GO TIME!

2. "Facts about Vitamin K Deficiency Bleeding," Centers for Disease Control and Prevention, last updated September 15, 2017, https://www.cdc.gov/ncbddd/vitamink/facts.html#ref.

3. Section on Breastfeeding, "Breastfeeding and the Use of Human Milk," *Pediatrics* 129, no. 3 (March 2012): e827–e841, https://doi.org/10.1542/peds.2011-3552.

4. Clair Barber et al., "The Safety of Formula Switching for Infants" (Poster, University of Virginia Children's Hospital 24th Annual Research Symposium, 2012), https://www.storebrandformula.com/Switching-Formulas-Store-Brand-Formula-Clinical-Study.pdf.

The researchers took sixty-seven infants who were formula-fed with "national" or name-brand formulas and switched them in three different ways. A third were switched to a generic "store-brand" formula, a third were switched to a different national brand, and a third were not switched at all. Parents did not know which group their infant was in. Researchers looked at spitting up, burping, gas, crying, and irritability before and after the change and found absolutely no differences in the kids switched to the store brand.

5. "Breastfeeding Report Card 2016: Progressing Toward National Breastfeeding Goals," Centers for Disease Control and Prevention, August 2016, https://www.cdc.gov/breastfeeding/pdf/2016 breastfeedingreportcard.pdf.

6. Task Force on Circumcision, "Circumcision Policy Statement.," *Pediatrics* 130, no. 3 (September 2012): 585–586, https://doi.org/10.1542/peds.2012-1989.

7. Melissa Buryk et al., "Efficacy of Neonatal Release of Ankyloglossia: A Randomized Trial," *Pediatrics* 128, no. 2 (August 2011): 280–288, https://doi.org/10.1542/peds.2011-0077.

In this study, newborns with trouble breastfeeding and evidence of *anterior* tongue-tie were assigned to two groups. Thirty babies got a frenotomy (a simple office procedure where the doctor clips the tongue-tie), and twenty-eight had a fake procedure where it was not clipped. Moms reported improvement in breastfeeding pain in both groups, but significantly more in the frenotomy group. Breastfeeding scores were markedly improved only in the frenotomy group.

TWO WEEKS

8. Robert Carpenter et al., "Bed sharing when parents do not smoke: is there a risk of SIDS? An individual level analysis of five major case-control studies," *BMJ Open* 3, no. 5 (May 2013): https://doi.org/10.1136/bmjopen-2012-002299.

This study looked at five quality studies comparing 1,472 SIDS cases with 4,679 controls. We already knew that smoking, alcohol use, and other drug use puts babies at risk of SIDS. This study was unique because it looked at babies who were breastfed with no parental substance use and no other risk factors. It included families of multiple races and socioeconomic classes. The researchers found that co-sleeping babies were *five times* more likely to die from SIDS when they were less than three months old. Smoking and alcohol use further increased this risk.

9. Denise G. Pitre and Amy Acker, "Accuracy of parents and health care professionals at estimating infant emesis volume," *Paediatrics & Child Health* 18, no. 1 (January 2013): 21–24, https://www.ncbi.nlm.nih.gov/pmc/articles/PMC3680267/.

Researchers in Canada recruited 271 caregivers and spilled different amounts of formula on baby blankets and pajamas. The caregivers had to guess the volumes that were spilled. Depending on the volume, their guesses were 130 percent to 275 percent of the actual amounts! That's a lot of simulated vomit.

10. Sung V et al., "*Lactobacillus reuteri* to treat infant colic: a meta-analysis." *Pediatrics* 141, no. 1 (January 2018): https://doi.org/10.1542/peds.2017-1811.

Many pediatricians have been recommending *Lactobacillus reuteri* for several years to help colicky babies and their desperate parents. The handful of studies looking at this were small and the results were somewhat mixed. This study in 2017 really put everything together. The authors combined four high-quality, double-blind, placebo-controlled trials that included a total of about 345 infants. They found that breastfed (but not formula-fed) infants receiving the probiotic were about twice as likely to have "treatment success" (defined as at least a 50 percent reduction in crying) at twenty-one days after starting the trial.

11. David Sas et al., "*Pseudomonas aeruginosa* septic shock secondary to 'Gripe Water' ingestion," *Pediatric Infectious Disease Journal* 23, no. 2 (February 2004): 176–177, https://doi.org/10.1097/01.inf.0000109722.53766.4f.

12. Tiffany Field, "Postpartum depression effects on early interactions, parenting, and safety practices: A review," *Infant Behavior & Development* 33, no. 1 (February 2010): 1–6, https://doi.org/10.1016/j.infbeh.2009.10.005.

VACCINES!

13. Brendan Nyhan et al., "Effective Messages in Vaccine Promotion: A Randomized Trial," *Pediatrics* 133, no. 4 (April 2014): 1–8, https://doi.org/10.1542/peds.2013-2365.

This was a humbling study that sent a few shockwaves across the pediatrics community. The authors assigned 1,759 parents to a control group or one of four intervention groups, which were given the following info to increase MMR (measles, mumps, rubella) vaccination rates:

1. Information from the CDC that shows no link between MMR and autism
2. A few paragraphs from the standard "Vaccine Information Sheet" about the dangers of measles
3. Pictures of sad-looking kids with illnesses prevented by the MMR vaccine
4. A dramatic story about a kid who almost died from measles

But none of the interventions worked. In fact, most of them actually decreased parents' intentions to vaccinate! And the scary pictures and stories actually increased parents' beliefs in harmful side effects from vaccines. What?!

14. "Vaccine Information Statements," Centers for Disease Control and Prevention, last updated July 6, 2017, https://www.cdc.gov/vaccines/hcp/vis/current-vis.html.

15. "Rotovirus in the U.S.," Centers for Disease Control and Prevention, last updated May 12, 2014, https://www.cdc.gov/rotavirus/surveillance.html.

16. Ramsay DS, Lewis M., "Developmental change in infant cortisol and behavioral response to inoculation," *Child Development* 65, no. 5 (October 1994):1491–1502, https://www.ncbi.nlm.nih.gov/pubmed/7982364.

17. Paul A. Offit et al., "Addressing Parents' Concerns: Do Multiple Vaccines Overwhelm or Weaken the Infant's Immune System?" *Pediatrics* 109, no. 1 (January 2002):124–129, https://doi.org/10.1542/peds.109.1.124.

18. Paul A. Offit and Rita K. Jew, "Addressing Parents' Concerns: Do Vaccines Contain Harmful Preservatives, Adjuvants, Additives, or Residuals?" *Pediatrics* 112, no. 6 (December 2003): 1394–1397, http://pediatrics.aappublications.org/content/112/6/1394.

19. Michael E. Pichichero et al., "Mercury concentrations and metabolism in infants receiving vaccines containing thimerosal: a descriptive study," *The Lancet* 360, no. 9347 (November 2002): 1737–1741, https://doi.org/10.1016/S0140-6736(02)11682-5.

TWO MONTHS

20. Farrah B. Lazare et al., "Rapid Resolution of Milk Protein Intolerance in Infancy," *Journal of Pediatric Gastroenterology and Nutrition* 59, no. 2 (August 2014): 215–217, https://doi.org/10.1097/MPG.0000000000000372.

21. Jack P. Shonkoff et al., "The Lifelong Effects of Early Childhood Adversity and Toxic Stress," *Pediatrics* 129, no. 1 (January 2002): e232–e246, https://doi.org/10.1542/peds.2011-2663.

22. Betty Hart and Todd R. Risley, "The Early Catastrophe: The 30 Million Word Gap by age 3," *American Educator* (Spring 2003): 4–9, https://www.aft.org/sites/default/files/periodicals/TheEarlyCatastrophe.pdf.

The researchers followed forty-two families in different socioeconomic groups from poverty to high income. They followed them monthly from the time their child was three months up until three years. They found huge discrepancies in the number of words that the different groups of kids heard—616 per hour in the poverty group versus 2,153 in the high-income group. Adding up all these hours yields the mind-blowing thirty-million word gap mentioned in the title of the article. There were also huge differences in the *type* of language the kids heard. High-income kids heard about six positive reinforcements for every negative one. The kids in the poverty group heard twice as many negative reinforcements as positive ones. Finally, they revisited twenty-nine of the families when the kids were in third grade. How many words they had heard correlated strongly with school performance in reading and language.

23. Frederick J. Zimmerman et al., "Associations between Media Viewing and Language Development in Children Under Age 2 Years," *The Journal of Pediatrics* 151, no. 4 (October 2007): 364–368, https://doi.org/10.1016/j.jpeds.2007.04.071.

This study done at the University of Washington surveyed 1,008 parents of kids between the ages of two and twenty-four months about how much time they spent watching "educational" baby videos like "Baby Einstein." The researchers found that for every hour kids spent watching educational videos, they learned about six to eight *fewer* new vocabulary words than kids who did not watch the videos. Kids who watched the videos scored about 10 percent lower on language skill tests compared with kids who did not watch the videos.

24. Roman Prymula et al., "Effect of prophylactic paracetamol administration at time of vaccination on febrile reactions and antibody responses in children: two open-label randomized controlled trials," *The Lancet* 374, no. 9698 (October 2009): 1139–1350, https://doi.org/10.1016/S0140-6736(09)61208-3.

This study looked at 459 healthy infants who were randomly assigned to either get acetaminophen every six to eight hours after receiving vaccines or to not get anything. Two outcomes were assessed. First, infants in the acetaminophen group had (not surprisingly) less fever than infants who received nothing. But only four of the kids, or less than 1 percent, had a very high fever of 104 or more. Second, infants who got acetaminophen formed fewer antibodies (the substance they store to fight off the illness if they ever come into contact with it) than the infants who got nothing.

FOUR MONTHS

25. Bee Wilson, *First Bite: How We Learn to Eat* (New York: Basic Books, 2015).

26. Thomas Walter et al., "Effectiveness of Iron-Fortified Infant Cereal in Prevention of Iron Deficiency Anemia," *Pediatrics* 91, no. 5 (May 1993): 976–982, http://pediatrics.aappublications.org/content/91/5/976.

27. Julie A. Mennella et al., "Prenatal and Postnatal Flavor Learning by Human Infants," *Pediatrics* 107, no. 6 (June 2001): E88, https://doi.org/10.1542/peds.107.6.e88.

The researchers in this study divided forty-six pregnant women into three groups: The first group drank carrot juice every day during pregnancy and then stopped after the birth, the second group breastfed and drank carrot juice every day only after the birth, and the third drank no carrot juice at any time. They then looked at their babies' reactions to eating carrot-flavored cereal after five months and found that the first two groups made fewer negative facial expressions. This is pretty cool. We have known for a long time that setting a good example of healthy eating makes babies more likely to eat better when they're older, but this study suggests that you can start that process before they're even born!

28. George Du Toit et al., "Randomized Trial of Peanut Consumption in Infants at Risk for Peanut Allergy," *The New England Journal of Medicine* 372, no. 9 (February 2015): 803–13, https://doi.org/10.1056/NEJMoa1414850.

This study, also known as the LEAP study (Learning Early About Peanut allergy), looked at 640 infants between the ages of four and eleven months at higher risk for peanut allergy (i.e., those with severe eczema or known egg allergy). Allergy testing made sure that they didn't already have an allergy. They were then split into two groups: half regularly ate peanut until age five, and half completely avoided it. The results were dramatic: 13.6 percent of the kids who avoided peanuts had allergy at age five versus only 1.9 percent of the kids who consumed them. That's an 86 percent reduction!

29. Maryse F. Bouchard et al., "Attention-Deficit/Hyperactivity Disorder and Urinary Metabolites of Organophosphate Pesticides," *Pediatrics* 125, no. 6 (June 2010): e1270–e1277, https://doi.org/10.1542/peds.2009-3058.

30. Mei Chen et al., "Residential Exposure to Pesticide During Childhood and Childhood Cancers: A Meta-Analysis," *Pediatrics* 136, no. 4 (October 2015): 719–729, https://doi.org/10.1542/peds.2015-0006.

31. Anna M. H. Price et al., "Five-Year Follow-up of Harms and Benefits of Behavioral Infant Sleep Intervention: Randomized Trial," *Pediatrics* 130, no. 4 (October 2012): 643–651, https://doi.org/10.1542/peds.2011-3467.

It's normal to worry about "crying it out"—particularly whether it will cause any long-term issues. This is a pretty good study that tried to answer that question. The researchers enrolled 225 seven-month-olds with sleep problems and then assigned some of them to sleep training. They followed the kids until six years old to see how they did. They found that the kids who were sleep trained did not differ at all in any measurement of their well-being. They also found improved sleep through age two years in the sleep-trained group. Moms did better in the sleep-trained group too, with better sleep and less depression through age two.

32. Sonya Lynne Cameron et al., "Healthcare professionals' and mothers' knowledge of, attitudes to and experiences with, Baby-Led Weaning: a content analysis study," *BMJ Open* 2, no. 6 (January 2012): https://doi.org/10.1136/bmjopen-2012-001542.

SIX MONTHS

33. Michael L. Macknin et al., "Symptoms Associated With Infant Teething: A Prospective Study," *Pediatrics* 105, no. 4 (April 2000): 747–752, https://doi.org/10.1542/peds.105.4.747.

This study followed 125 healthy children from four months old to twelve months old. Parents recorded multiple temperatures and the presence or absence of eighteen different symptoms every day. They also recorded every tooth eruption so the symptoms could be correlated. They found that the following symptoms were associated with teething:

- Increased biting and drooling
- Gum rubbing and sucking
- Irritability and wakefulness
- Ear rubbing
- Facial rash
- Decreased appetite for solid foods

The symptoms were not very strong. None of them occurred in more than 35 percent of teething infants. Teething did not seem to cause very loose stools, significant congestion, severe sleep disturbances, fevers over 102 degrees, or rashes on other parts of the body.

34. Committee on Children with Disabilities, "The Treatment of Neurologically Impaired Children Using Patterning," *Pediatrics* 104, no. 5 (November 1999): 1149–1151, https://doi.org/10.1542/peds.104.5.1149.

35. Committee on Injury and Poison Prevention, "Injuries Associated With Infant Walkers.," *Pediatrics* 108, no. 3 (September 2001): 790–792, https://doi.org/10.1542/peds.108.3.790.

36. Siegel AC, Burton RV, "Effects of baby walkers on motor and mental development in human infants.," *Journal of Developmental & Behavioral Pediatrics* 20, no. 5 (October 1999): 355–361, https://www.ncbi.nlm.nih.gov/pubmed/10533994.

NINE MONTHS

37. "Choking—infant under 1 year," MedlinePlus, U.S. National Library of Medicine, last updated December 21, 2017, https://www.nlm.nih.gov/medlineplus/ency/article/000048.htm.

U.S. National Library of Medicine website with choking guidelines for children under one year old.

38. Gillman MW et al., "Family dinner and diet quality among older children and adolescents," *Archives of Family Medicine* 9, no. 3 (March 2000): 235–240, https://www.ncbi.nlm.nih.gov/pubmed/10728109.

This study looked at 8,677 girls and 7,525 boys ages nine to fourteen. They found that 17 percent ate dinner with their families never or hardly at all, 40 percent most of the time, and 43 percent some of the time. They found that kids who tended to eat with their families ate significantly more fruits and vegetables, less saturated fats, less fried foods, and more vitamins.

39. Beals DE, "Sources of support for learning words in conversation: evidence from mealtimes," *Journal of Child Language* 24, no. 3 (October 1997): 673–694, https://www.ncbi.nlm.nih.gov/pubmed/9519590.

This study looked at the recordings of 160 mealtime conversations of sixty-eight different families in the Boston area with three- to five-year-old children. Obviously dinnertime is a great time to talk, but this study looked at the *type* of words in those conversations. They found that rare words (those not on a list of 3,000 "common" words) were used a lot more often during mealtime conversations than at other times. About two-thirds of the time the parents said the words in a way that helped the child figure out the meaning (by giving some context or directly explaining the word, for example). The more rare words the kids heard in this way, the better their vocabulary scores were at ages five and seven. Knowing "rare words" is also important for early reading.

TWELVE MONTHS

40. "Raw Milk Questions and Answers," Centers for Disease Control and Prevention, last updated September 1, 2017, www.cdc.gov/foodsafety/rawmilk/raw-milk-questions-and-answers.html.

FIFTEEN MONTHS

41. Julie Crandall, "Poll: Most Approve of Spanking Kids," ABC News, accessed January 16, 2018, http://abcnews.go.com/US/story?id=90406.

42. Catherine, A. Taylor et al., "Mothers' Spanking of 3-Year-Old Children and Subsequent Risk of Children's Aggressive Behavior," *Pediatrics* 125, no. 5 (May 2010): e1057–e1065, https://doi.org/10.1542/peds.2009-2678.

This study looked at 2,461 moms from twenty states who enrolled in a big "cohort" upon the birth of their children. Researchers have therefore been able to follow the group throughout childhood to collect multiple kinds of data. Moms were asked about spanking at age three and then were asked how aggressive their children were at age five. Kids who were spanked frequently (more than twice per month) had one and a half times more aggressive behavior at age five. The researchers controlled for things like race, economic status, domestic violence, and substance abuse, so they felt confident that the changes were due to spanking.

43. Murray A. Straus and Mallie J. Paschall, "Corporal Punishment by Mothers and Development of Children's Cognitive Ability: A Longitudinal Study of Two Nationally Representative Age Cohorts," *Journal of Aggression, Maltreatment, and Trauma* 18, no. 5 (July 2009): 459–483, https://doi.org/10.1080/10926770903035168.

44. Akemi Tomoda et al., "Reduced prefrontal cortical gray matter volume in young adults exposed to harsh corporal punishment," *NeuroImage* 47, no. 2 (August 2009): T66–T71, https://doi.org/10.1016/j.neuroimage.2009.03.005.

EIGHTEEN MONTHS

45. Deborah L. Christensen et al., "Prevalence and Characteristics of Autism Spectrum Disorder Among Children Aged 8 Years—Autism and Developmental Disabilities Monitoring Network, 11 Sites, United States, 2012," *MMWR Surveillance Summaries* 65, no. 3 (April 2016): 1–23, https://doi.org/10.15585/mmwr.ss6503a1.

46. Mark DeBoer et al., "Sugar-Sweetened Beverages and Weight Gain in 2- to 5-Year-Old Children," *Pediatrics* 132, no. 3 (September 2013): 413–420, https://doi.org/10.1542/peds.2013-0570.

This study looked at "sugar-sweetened beverage" (soda and juice) consumption of 9,600 children aged two to five years followed in the Early Childhood Longitudinal Survey Birth Cohort (a group of kids followed from birth as a way of doing lots of interesting research). It found that kids who consumed more sugar-sweetened beverages were 40 percent more likely to be obese by ages four and five!

47. Robert H. Lustig et al., "Public health: The toxic truth about sugar," *Nature* 482, no. 7383 (February 2012): 27–29, https://doi.org/10.1038/482027a.

48. R. Bethene Ervin et al., "Consumption of Added Sugar Among U.S. Children and Adolescents, 2005–2008," Centers for Disease Control and Prevention, *NCHS Data Brief*, no. 87 (March 2012), https://www.cdc.gov/nchs/data/databriefs/db87.pdf.

49. Timothy R. Schum et al., "Sequential Acquisition of Toilet-Training Skills: A Descriptive Study of Gender and Age Differences in Normal Children," *Pediatrics* 109, no. 3 (March 2002): E48, https://doi.org/10.1542/peds.109.3.e48.

This study followed 267 children aged fourteen to forty-two months at four Milwaukee pediatric offices. They collected weekly surveys from the children's parents on toilet-training behaviors for a year or more. First they looked at factors that predicted readiness. Girls began showing interest in using the potty at an average of twenty-four months vs twenty-six for boys. Girls were staying dry for two hours and indicating that they had to use the potty at twenty-six months vs. twenty-nine for boys. The average age for starting to stay dry throughout the day (fully potty trained) was thirty-two and a half months for girls and thirty-five for boys.

TWO YEARS

50. Daniela J. Owen et al., "The Effect of Praise, Positive Nonverbal Response, Reprimand, and Negative Nonverbal Response on Child Compliance: A Systematic Review," *Clinical Child and Family Psychology Review* 15, no. 4 (December 2012): 364–385, https://doi.org/10.1007/s10567-012-0120-0.

There are many studies on discipline, but what's great about this study is that it looked at all of them! Well, forty-one of them. Individual studies can often contradict one another, so a review study like this is helpful at identifying trends. The studies included "negative" discipline such as time-outs and taking away privileges, and "positive" discipline such as praise and hugs. The authors made it clear that they did not consider studies that used harsh words or methods. The negative discipline was associated with better compliance in *every study* they looked at. Pretty impressive.

51. AAP Council on Communications and Media, "Media and Young Minds," *Pediatrics* 138, no. 5 (November 2016), https://doi.org/10.1542/peds.2016-2591.

52. Elizabeth M. Cespedes et al., "Television Viewing, Bedroom Television, and Sleep Duration From Infancy to Mid-Childhood," *Pediatrics* 133, no. 5 (May 2014): e1163–e1171, https://doi.org/10.1542/peds.2013-3998.

53. Ling-Yi Lin et al., "Effects of television exposure on developmental skills among young children," *Infant Behavior and Development* 38 (February 2015): 20–26, https://doi.org/10.1016/j.infbeh.2014.12.005.

54. Edward L. Swing et al., "Television and Video Game Exposure and the Development of Attention Problems," *Pediatrics* 126, no. 2 (August 2010): 214–221, https://doi.org/10.1542/peds.2009-1508.

55. Yalda T. Uhls et al., "Five days at outdoor education camp without screens improves preteen skills with nonverbal emotional cues," *Computers in Human Behavior* 39 (October 2014): 387–392, https://doi.org/10.1016/j.chb.2014.05.036.

56. Daniel R. Anderson and Tiffany A. Pempek, "Television and Very Young Children," *American Behavioral Scientist* 48, no. 5 (January 2005): 505–522, https://doi.org/10.1177/0002764204271506.

57. Marie Evans Schmidt et al., "The Effects of Background Television on the Toy Play Behavior of Very Young Children," *Child Development* 79, no. 4 (July 2008): 1137–1151, https://doi.org/10.1111/j.1467-8624.2008.01180.x.

58. Heather L. Kirkorian et al., "The Impact of Background Television on Parent-Child Interaction," *Child Development* 80, no. 5 (September 2009): 1350–1359, https://doi.org/10.1111/j.1467-8624.2009.01337.x.

59. Kelly L. Schmitt and Daniel R. Anderson, "Television and Reality: Toddlers' Use of Visual Information from Video to Guide Behavior," *Media Psychology* 4, no. 1 (2002): 51–76, https://doi.org/10.1207/S1532785XMEP0401_03.

Multiple studies suggest that young kids can imitate what they see on TV but do not really learn. This was an interesting study in which the researchers looked at three groups of kids: two-year-olds, two-and-a-half-year-olds, and three-year-olds. The kids watched a toy being placed in an adjacent room and then had to either find it or put it in the same place. Half of the kids watched the toy being hidden through a window, and half watched it on a screen. At all ages, kids did great when watching directly through the window, getting it right over 85 percent of the time. But when watching on TV, two-year-olds got it right only 25 percent of the time (about what you'd expect from chance) and two-and-a-half year-olds got it right a little over 50 percent of the time. By three, the kids were just about as good at the task whether watching it directly or on the TV.

60. Tovah P. Klein, "Why You Can't Teach a Toddler to Share," *Tips on Life and Love* (blog), March 21, 2014, http://www.tipsonlifeandlove.com/parenting/why-you-cant-teach-a-toddler-to-share.

THREE TO FOUR YEARS

61. Brie A. Moore et al., "Brief Report: Evaluating the Bedtime Pass Program for Child Resistance to Bedtime—A Randomized, Controlled Trial," *Journal of Pediatric Psychology* 32, no.3 (April 2007): 283–287, https://doi.org/10.1093/jpepsy/jsl025.

This study looked at nineteen three- to six-year-old children with significant bedtime problems who were assigned to a treatment group that got a bedtime pass or a control group that didn't get any intervention. Parents were trained to allow their kids to use the bedtime pass once per night to get out of their bed for a quick visit, hug, drink of water, etc. After that, parents ignored requests to get out of bed. After just nine days of treatment, kids who got the bedtime pass showed a shorter time falling asleep, less crying out in the night, and less leaving their room. Also, these benefits were maintained to a high degree at a three-month follow-up.

62. John Medina, *Brain Rules For Baby*, (Seattle: Pear Press, 2010).

63. Ramey CT et al., *Early Learning, Later Success: The Abecedarian Study*, Executive Summary, (Chapel Hill, NC: Frank Porter Graham Child Development Center, University of North Carolina, 1999), http://fpg.unc.edu/sites/fpg.unc.edu/files/resources/reports-and-policy-briefs/EarlyLearningLaterSuccess_1999.pdf.

The Abecedarian Project was an experiment conducted in North Carolina more than forty years ago. The researchers enrolled 111 infants who were "at risk" of poor outcomes due to socioeconomic factors such as family income and maternal education. Half of the kids were given high-quality childcare starting as infants. This included preschool until age five with a low teacher-to-child ratio of one to six. Half of the kids served as "controls" who got good health care, social services, and nutritional help, but no extra help with childcare or preschool. Then they followed these kids at regular intervals until they were thirty!

The kids who got good childcare and preschool did better in a lot of ways. At age twenty-one they were nearly two grade levels higher in reading and over one grade level higher in math. Their IQs were an average of 4.4 points higher. Forty-two percent were still in some kind of school compared with only 20 percent of controls. Forty-seven percent were performing skilled jobs compared with only 27 percent of controls.

64. Anna C. Roby and Evan Kidd, "The referential communication skills of children with imaginary companions," *Developmental Science* 11, no. 4 (July 2008): 531–540, https://doi.org/10.1111/j.1467-7687.2008.00699.x.

65. Eva V. Hoff, "Imaginary Companions, Creativity, and Self-Image in Middle Childhood," *Creativity Research Journal* 17, no. 2–3 (2005): 167–180, https://doi.org/10.1080/10400419.2005.9651477.

CASES

66. "Allergy Statistics," American Academy of Allergy, Asthma, and Immunology, accessed January 16, 2018, www.aaaai.org/about-aaaai/newsroom/allergy-statistics.

67. Jackson KD et al., "Trends in allergic conditions among children: United States, 1997–2011," *NCHS Data Brief*, no. 121 (May 2013), https://www.ncbi.nlm.nih.gov/pubmed/23742874.

68. Ruchi S. Gupta et al., "Factors associated with reported food allergy tolerance among US children," *Annals of Allergy, Asthma & Immunology* 111, no. 3 (September 2013): 194–198, https://doi.org/10.1016/j.anai.2013.06.026.

69. Amir A. Azari and Neal P. Barney, "Conjunctivitis: A Systematic Review of Diagnosis and Treatment," *JAMA* 310, no. 16 (October 2013): 1721–1729, https://doi.org/10.1001/jama.2013.280318.

70. Ian M. Paul et al., "Effect of Honey, Dextromethorphan, and No Treatment on Nocturnal Cough and Sleep Quality for Coughing Children and Their Parents," *Archives of Pediatrics and Adolescent Medicine* 161, no. 12 (December 2007): 1140–1146, https://doi.org/10.1001/archpedi.161.12.1140.

This was a simple but effective study that tried to answer the burning question of "What can I do to help my child's cough at night?" The authors looked at 105 kids from ages two to eighteen with nighttime coughs due to viruses. They divided the kids into three groups: no treatment, treatment with pure honey, and treatment with honey-flavored dextromethorphan (the most common ingredient in cough syrups). Then they surveyed parents the following day. The kids who got honey coughed significantly less and had fewer symptoms overall than the no treatment group, while the kids who got cough syrup did not do better than the no-treatment group. The improvement was modest, but my takeaways from this study were to avoid cough syrup since it doesn't work anyway, and that honey is a safe and soothing thing to give your child when he's struggling with nighttime cough.

71. Caleb K. King et al., "Managing Acute Gastroenteritis Among Children: Oral Rehydration, Maintenance, and Nutritional Therapy," Centers for Disease Control and Prevention, *Morbidity and Mortality Weekly Report*, November 21, 2003: 1–16, https://www.cdc.gov/mmwr/preview/mmwrhtml/rr5216a1.htm.

Index

G

L

—

M

—

N

—

About the Author

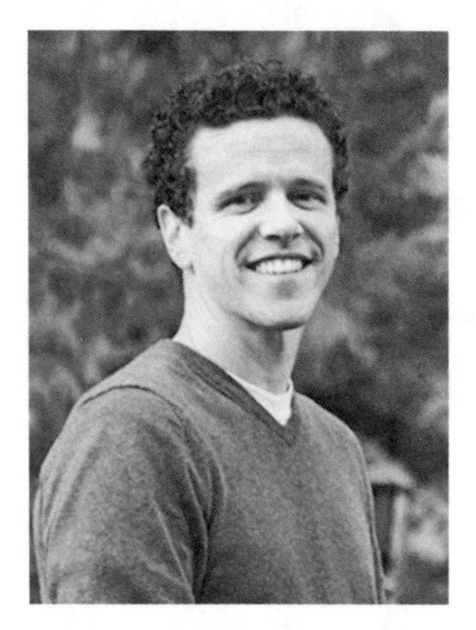

LUKE VOYTAS is a board-certified pediatrician living in Portland, Oregon. He works full time at Evergreen Pediatrics in Vancouver, Washington, where he sees kids from birth to age eighteen. He has also served as Chair of Pediatrics at Peacehealth Southwest Medical Center and teaches family medicine residents. He did his undergraduate work at Duke University, medical school at Washington University in St. Louis, and pediatrics residency at Children's Hospital Los Angeles.

He has two wonderful kids of his own, ages six and eight. His wife is a pediatrician too, and the one that their friends usually call for parenting advice. In his free time, you can find him hiking, playing shuffleboard, shivering on the Oregon coast, running, and complaining about injuries that prevent him from running.

Learn more at BeyondtheCheckup.com.